Practical Herbs 2

Henriette Kress

Front cover: Lemon beebalm (Monarda citriodora).
Back cover: Annual malope or mallowwort (Malope trifida).

Disclaimer
The purpose of this book is solely informational and educational. The information and suggestions in this book are not intended to replace the advice or treatments given by health professionals. The author and publisher have made every effort to present accurate information. However, they shall be neither responsible nor liable for any problem that may arise from information in this book.

First published in Finland in 2013.

This edition published 2018 by

Aeon Books Ltd
12 New College Parade
Finchley Road
London
NW3 5EP

British Library Cataloguing in Publication Data

A C.I.P. for this book is available from the British Library

ISBN-13: 978-1-91159-758-2

www.aeonbooks.co.uk

PREFACE

In 2000 and 2001 I wrote two herb books in Finnish. They were quite good. Both have been out of print for years and are utterly unobtainable: you won't find them in any used book stores in Finland.

Because people kept asking me for them, I wrote Practical Herbs (in Finnish) in 2010, translating it into English in 2011. This was 150 pages of dense text about herbs. As a new mom, I simply didn't have the time to make that book more comprehensive.

But I had more to say about herbs. In 2012, I wrote Practical Herbs 2 in Finnish. You hold my English translation in your hands.

This book provides in-depth information on 20 herbs, green powder, herbal honeys, a few inconveniences, and herbal uses for a few common vegetables.

I'm happy with this book. I hope you will be, too!

ACKNOWLEDGMENTS

I thank everyone who asked questions and shared their experiences with me during my lectures. I also thank my wonderful clients, who have helped me gain experience using herbs to treat a variety of disorders as they manifest in different types of people, and all the herbalists and herbal hobbyists who have shared their knowledge, experiences, and tips in online forums, blogs, and websites.

I'd also like to thank those who proofread and offered suggestions on this text.

I reserve my most heartfelt thanks for my teachers, now deceased—my grandmother E. Brennecke and the herbalist Michael Moore.

I wish you much joy in the world of herbs!

Henriette Kress
October 2013

A new edition, enjoy!

Henriette Kress, November 2020

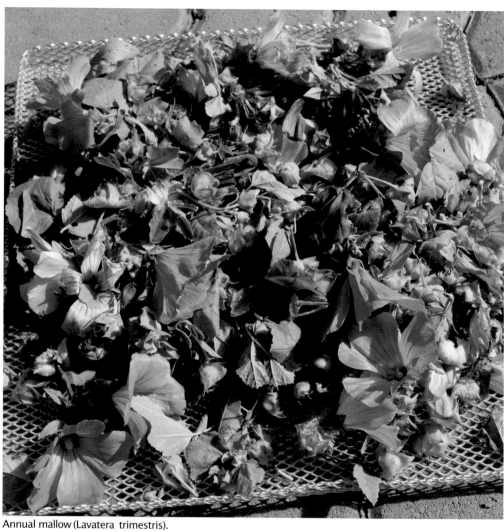

Annual mallow (Lavatera trimestris).

TABLE OF CONTENTS

THE BASICS: RECIPES

HERBAL SYRUP

Herbal syrups are runny. They preserve the herb for later use.

A good herbal syrup contains enough sugar to ensure that it won't spoil or grow mold. It also contains enough water that it won't crystallize easily.

How to make an herbal syrup

1 quart (1 l) water
1 cup (250 ml) fresh herb material
  or 0.5-0.7 ounces (15-20 g) dried
    aboveground parts
  or 1 cup (250 ml) fresh or dried roots or
    bark, in smallish pieces
13 ounces (425 g) granulated sugar

Put the herb in a saucepan and cover it with the water. Bring to a boil and simmer covered or uncovered 15-25 minutes. Strain. (For a stronger syrup, add more herb to the same liquid, simmer another 15-25 minutes, and strain.)

Add sugar to 3/4 cup (200 ml) of the strained liquid, set the heat as low as possible, and stir until the sugar has dissolved.

Pour the syrup into glass jars, seal with a tight-fitting lid, and label (example: "Herbal syrup, peppermint and thyme, June 2021. 1 tsp. as needed for cough.").

Keep your syrup in the fridge.

For detailed syrup-making instructions, see the earlier volume Practical Herbs.

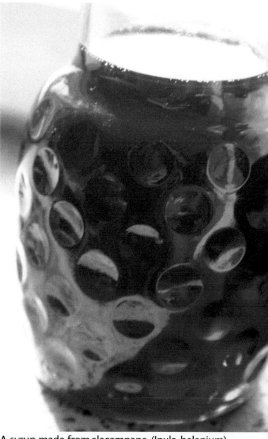

A syrup made from elecampane (Inula helenium) and roselle (Hibiscus sabdariffa). The roselle makes the syrup red and tart.

1

HERBAL HONEY

Herbal honeys are great for coughs.

Use peppermint, beebalm, hyssop, elecampane, angelica, garlic, onion, basil, ginger, chamomile, thyme, sage, or other strong-flavored herbs—alone or in blends.

How to make an herbal honey

fresh or dried herbs, chopped fine
organic honey

Fresh herb: Fill a jar halfway with chopped herbs or to one-fourth with chopped roots.

Dried herb: Fill a jar to one-fourth with herb matter.

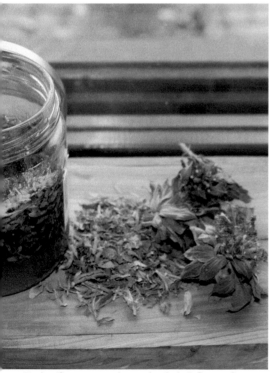

Herbs (for instance, lemon beebalm) float in honey.

Fill jar to the brim with honey and seal with a tight-fitting lid.

Invert the jar every few days to thoroughly mix the herb with the honey.

The honey is done in 2-6 weeks.

Strain the honey, if you like. If you prefer to leave the honey as it is, note that the herb will float to the top.

Take a spoonful of honey or honeyed herb as needed to soothe coughs, scratchy throats, and the like.

Herbal tea honey

½cup (100 ml) strong herbal tea
½cup (100 ml) organic honey

First, make a strong herbal tea:
1-3 tablespoons dried or fresh herbs
1 cup (250 ml) boiling water

Pour boiling water over the herb, steep for 20 minutes, and strain.

Dissolve the honey in the hot tea, pour into a jar, and refrigerate.

Take a teaspoon as needed.

Because this blend can ferment even in the fridge, don't seal the jar tightly. And use it up quickly, if it does ferment.

Garlic honey

cloves of two garlic bulbs
organic honey

Peel and finely chop the cloves. Pour them into a jar and cover with honey. Let steep at least overnight.

Take a teaspoon as needed for coughs, colds, or the flu.

Share your garlic honey, so that you're not the only one with garlic breath!

HERBAL SUGAR

Although there are no medicinal uses for herbal sugars, they can be useful in cooking.

Make your sugars using dried herbs. Otherwise, you'll end up with a sticky mess that attracts flies and wasps.

How to make an herbal sugar

1 cup (250 ml) granulated sugar
½–1 cup (100–250 ml) dried powdered
   herbs such as blackcurrant (Ribes nigrum)
   leaf, rose petals, or peppermint

Mix.

Use light sugars. The strong flavor of darker sugars can overpower even the strongest peppermint.

Try your peppermint sugar in rhubarb pie. Delicious!

Vanilla sugar

In Finland, instead of vanilla extract we cook with vanilla sugar—or its artificial alternative, vanillin sugar. Homemade vanilla sugar beats the artificial versions hands down, and it's very easy to make:

1 vanilla bean
sugar

Cut your vanilla bean into pieces short enough to fit into a ½–1 cup (100–250 ml) jar. Cover it with sugar, screw on the lid, and leave in room temperature for 4–6 weeks.

Add more sugar to the jar as you use it up. If you use a lot of vanilla sugar, keep two jars going—one in use and one steeping.

One vanilla bean is good for years of vanilla sugar.

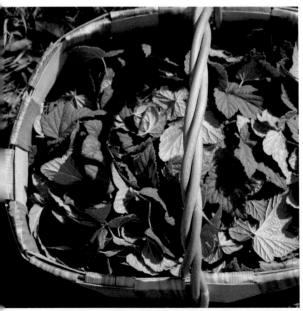

Blackcurrant (Ribes nigrum) leaf makes a tasty herbal sugar.

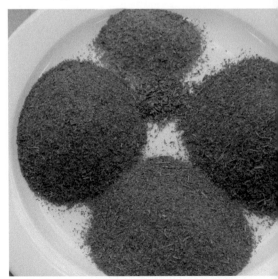

Green powder in progress—celery leaf, stinging nettle (Urtica dioica), bur-marigold (Bidens spp.), carrot leaf, and a little thyme in the middle.

GREEN POWDER

Green powders are a great way to add mineral-dense vegetable greens to your food.

Although it's made from the green parts of plants, you can also add more colorful parts. Spice it up with small amounts of strong-flavored herbs.

Grind your chosen materials into a powder and use the powder in your cooking, or add a spoonful or two to your food.

Make your green powder in small batches, in case the result isn't as delicious as you'd hoped.

Take a lot of herb material, such as

• nettle leaf, kale, bur-marigold(Bidens spp.)
• parsley, lovage, celery leaf
• carrot greens
• various mallows
• other mild-tasting plants

Add a few of these for flavor:

• spicy: thyme, basil, marjoram, oregano, beebalm, rosemary, chamomile, blackcurrant leaf, angelica leaf
• anise/licorice: sweet cicely (Myrrhis odorata), aniseed, anise-y giant hyssops (Agastache spp.), goutweed leaf (Aegopodium spp.)
• lemony: lemon balm, lemon catnip, lemon grass, lemon thyme
• minty: peppermint, mountainmint (Pycnanthemum spp.)
• sweet: rose petals or lavender
• salty: various seaweeds
• bitter: dandelion leaf, burdock leaf, horehound, the lower leaf of goldenrod

• astringent: willowherb (Epilobium spp.), birch leaf, raspberry leaf, lady's mantle leaf, cinquefoil leaf, strawberry leaf
• oniony: onion greens, chives greens, garlic greens, garlic mustard greens (Alliaria petiolata)

Or experiment with others you like.

If you have them on hand, you can also add powdered berries to your blend. Mild berries include rosehip, hawthorn berries, and bilberry. Blackcurrant, cranberry, and lingonberry are very sour.

Various spicy roots can also enhance a green powder—for instance, calamus root (Acorus calamus), angelica root, or ginger.

How to make a green powder

Grind the dried plant parts in a blender (or a coffee grinder, for small batches), and then rub the powder through a sieve. Set aside any parts too large to go through the sieve and add them to your next blender batch.

Store your green powder in glass jars with tight-fittinglids. Label, for instance: "Minty green powder, June 2021."

Add a few tablespoons of green powder to soups, stews, and similar, or sprinkle a spoonful or two on the food on your plate.

HERBAL SALT

The easiest way to make an herbal salt is to add salt to a spicy green powder.

You can also make a green powder blend just for your herbal salt. For that, you'll need a lot of parsley, lovage, or celery leaf; some onion greens or dried onions; a little of a strong-tasting culinary herb, and other plant parts to taste.

How to make an herbal salt

2 ounces (50 g) dried herb (fresh herbs contain too much water)

½ ounce (12 g) fine dry salt (coarse sea salt is usually too damp to use for herbal salts)

You might feel tempted to use a mug to measure your mix. Don't. Two cups of green powder to half a cup of salt will make for an oversalted mix.

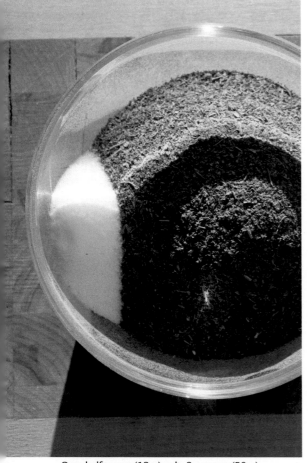

One-half ounce (12 g) salt, 2 ounces (50 g) powdered herb.

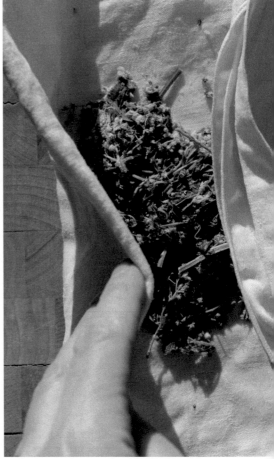

An herbal poultice made with meadowsweet.

HERBAL POULTICES AND COMPRESSES

Poultices (wraps) and compresses (fomentations) are similar in that both involve herbs heated in water.

To make a compress, you dip a cloth in hot liquid and apply it to the affected body part. To make a poultice, you remove the hot herb mass from the water, fold it inside a cloth, and apply it to the aching part.

Good herbs to use for compresses and poultices include

- for pain: meadowsweet, balsam poplar buds, willow, and (especially for joint pain) horsetail
- to increase local blood supply: ginger, mustard, angelica, yarrow, horsetail, and (especially for hemorrhoids) mullein
- for bruises, strains and sprains: St. John's wort, calendula, hyssop, mullein, chamomile, horsetail, yarrow, sweet clover (Melilotus officinalis)

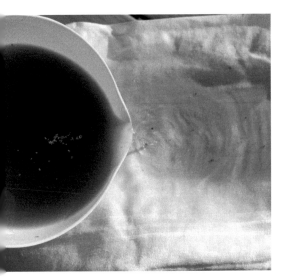

- for irritated skin, eczema, itch: rose petals, mallow, plantain (Plantago spp.), chickweed, burdock, calendula, chamomile
- for menstrual or gut pain and for coughs: oregano, angelica, the mints, catnip, sage, beebalm, thyme, basil, chamomile, fennel, aniseed

Cold compresses are also effective. Some lemon juice in cool water can be applied to the calves, for example, to help lower a high fever.

How to make a poultice or compress

1–2 cups (250–500 ml) finely chopped aboveground plant parts
or ½–1 cup (100–200 ml) finely chopped roots
1 quart (1 l) boiling water

Add water and herb to a pan, bring to a boil, lower heat and simmer 10–20 minutes. Strain and cool until just skin-comfortable.

Compress: Dip a towel or rag in the tea, and squeeze out excess liquid. Put the moist, hot cloth on the hurt spot, cover it with a dry towel, and leave it there 20–30 minutes.

Poultice: Fold your hot moist herb into a towel or rag. Press the poultice onto the hurt spot and cover with a dry towel. Keep it in place 20–30 minutes.

Don't apply a poultice or compress more often than twice a day, or for more than 40 minutes at a time.

A towel moistened with hot, strong meadowsweet tea makes a good compress.

6

HERBAL OILS AND SALVES

For detailed instructions for making herbal oils and salves (ointments), see the earlier volume, Practical Herbs.

How to make an herbal oil

2 cups (500 ml) oil
fresh or dried herbs

Pour water into a saucepan. Suspend a metal bowl over the water so its sides don't touch the pan (three untreated bamboo chopsticks work well for this).

Pour oil into the bowl.

Cut your fresh herbs into 1-inch lengths (2–3 cm), or crush your dried herb. Add as much herb material as you can while keeping it completely covered with oil.

Bring the water to a boil, and then lower the heat to keep the water at a simmer. Add water as needed to keep the pan from boiling dry.

Leave your oil on your water bath 1½–2 hours.

A bain–marie—a bowl in a pan. The herb is calendula.

Lift the bowl off the pan and let the oil cool for 30 minutes. Then wipe the bowl's sides and rim of the bowl and strain the oil into another clean vessel.

Dried herb: Pour it into a bottle, cap tightly, and label (example: "Herbal oil: olive oil, dried meadowsweet, calendula. August 2021").

Fresh herb: Let the water separate from the oil and then pour it off.

Pour the strained oil into a wide–mouthed jar and let it settle in a corner (sunny, for St. John's wort; shady, for other herbs) 4–7 days—that is, until the oil clears. Pour the oil carefully off the bottom muck, bottle, and label (example: "Herbal oil, sesame oil, fresh St. John's wort, July 2021").

How to make an herbal salve

2 cups (400 ml) herbal oil
2.7 ounces (55 g) beeswax

Heat the oil in a bain–marie or double-boiler.

If your beeswax is in thin sheets (1–2 mm), tear it into strips and add to the heated oil. If you have beeswax buttons, add them whole.

Keep the water at a full boil, or your beeswax won't melt. Over-stirring cools the wax and keeps it from melting.

Your salve is ready to pour when the wax has melted completely into the oil. Wipe the underside of your oil bowl, especially the rim, and then carefully pour your salve into small jars.

Put lids and labels on the jars only after the salve has set and cooled completely.

HERBAL ENERGETICS

I include in this volume's plant sections two new descriptors—"Taste" and "Energetics."

Energetics involves using your own five senses to learn about herbs and determine how to use them. Incorporating a knowledge of basic herbal polarities makes it easier to get familiar with new herbs when you encounter them.

People and problems can also be divided by these polarities.

HOT AND COLD

The more important pairing in herbal energetics is hot–cold or the milder warm–cool.

You can classify a lot of plants this way, but some are neutral in heat.

Of the liquids, alcohol is hot, vinegar is cool, and oil, syrup, and water are neutral.

Warming plants

Hot plants include
chili, garlic, pepper, ginger, wasabi, mustard, horseradish, and even the flowering tops of beebalms in hot summers.

Warm plants include
common culinary herbs such as fennel, cinnamon, cardamom, basil, and thyme, as well as, for instance, catnip, hyssop, raw onion, elecampane, and angelica.

Warm

Aromatic or spicy herbs are energetically warm. Warm herbs speed up the metabolism and increase blood circulation.

Most culinary herbs and spices are warm, but you'll find warm herbs beyond the kitchen garden, as well.

At the far end of warm, you'll find plants so hot they'll produce blisters if held against unprotected skin for a length of time. Diluting them in teas, baths, and oils tames them somewhat.

Hot–and cold–neutral plants include
willowherb, cinquefoil, and raspberry leaf.

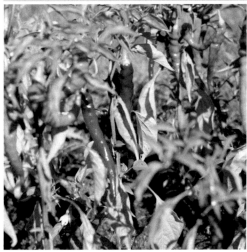

Very warming: chili pepper (Capsicum frutescens 'De Cayenne').

8

Cool

Very juicy or mucilaginous plants are cool. So are sour and bitter plants. Note: sour (lemon) isn't the same as bitter (dandelion or hops).

Some bitter herbs are also aromatic. They can be cool or warm or both at once.

Cool herbs calm or slow metabolism. Although bitter herbs enhance the flow of digestive juices, overusing them without adding warming herbs can in fact slow and impair your digestion.

Cold, of course, lies at the far end of cool. Cold plants slow the metabolism to the point of stagnation: instead of enhancing the digestion, they constipate. Or, in the case of too much coffee, your inner ear may become congested and you may acquire tinnitus and find it difficult to hear.

Cooling plants

Mucilaginous plants include
mallows, violets, plantain seeds (Plantago), bur-marigold, chia seed, aloe (the inner part of the leaf), flax seed, and boiled onions.

Juicy plants include
cucumber, chickweed, and jewelweed (Impatiens).

Bitter plants include
barberry (Berberis), dandelion, chicory, grapefruit, sage, hops, cocoa and coffee.

Sour plants include
lemon, grapefruit, and other citrus fruits, cranberry, lingonberry, strawberry, and raspberry.

Cooling and warming plants

Aromatic and bitter plants include
angelica, mugwort, southernwood, elecampane, citrus peel, sage, coffee, and juniper berries.

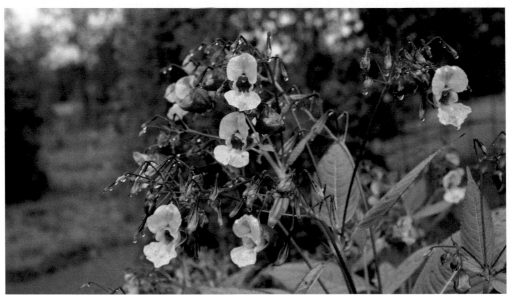

Cooling: Indian or Himalayan balsam (Impatiens glandulifera) in flower.

9

DRY AND MOIST

The other pairing in herbal energetics is dry-moist. It's a good idea to divide these further into watery and oily.

Some plants are neutral in dryness.

Of the liquids, oils, honeys, and syrups are moist. Alcohols are dry. Water is neutral.

Dry

Most warm or bitter plants are dry.

So are astringent plants: they remove surface water from mucous membranes, leaving them drier than before. They can be moist from a whole-body point of view, though, if they stop liquids leaving the body, as with diarrhea or drooling.

Plants that enhance the secretion of liquids are dry. These include diuretics (which make you pee), or plants that enhance secretion of sweat, milk, mucus, bile, or saliva, which dries the body.

Plants that address constipation or cause diarrhea are also dry.

Drying: oak leaf (Quercus robur).

Drying plants

Astringent plants include
oak leaf, alder cone, willowherb, cinquefoil, raspberry leaf, avens (Geum), geraniums, and black tea.

Diuretic plants include
birch leaf, nettle, goldenrod, horsetail, burdock, and dandelion.

Sweat-enhancing plants include
hot plants and hot sage tea.

Mucus-stimulators include
hot plants.

Milk-enhancers include
nettle, caraway, fennel, dill, aniseed, willowherb, and hot sage tea.

Sialagogues (which make you drool) include
echinacea, elecampane, spilanthes, and bitter plants.

Bile-enhancers include
bitter plants.

Purging plants (which make you poo) include
buckthorn(Frangula, Rhamnus), senna, and prune.

Emetics (which make you vomit) include
ipecac and lobelia.

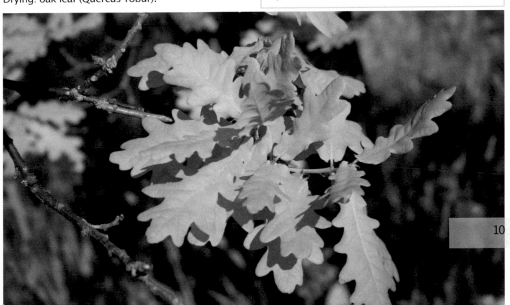

Moist

Moist plants slow a body's fluid loss.

Juicy or mucilaginous plants are moist in water.

Very oily or greasy plants are moist in fats.

Most herbs are either aromatic (hot and dry), bitter (cool and dry), mildly astringent (dry) or mucilaginous (moist). I can't think of any moisture–neutral plants.

Moist plants add to a body's moisture. They help with dryness—dry tissues, dry people.

CONDITIONS

Cold conditions take a long time to resolve. They can linger for weeks, months or even years.

Hot conditions are intense but resolve quickly.

Damp conditions ooze, dry conditions itch or flake.

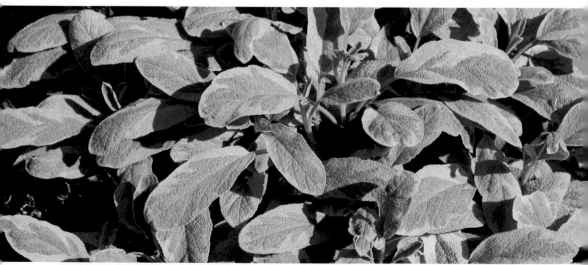

Warming, cooling, drying, moistening: sage is an aromatic bitter herb that can promote or reduce sweat and milk secretion.

APPLYING HERBAL ENERGETICS

Give warming and heating herbs to "cold" people—who walk around in sweaters when everyone else is in shorts and T-shirts—and to pale, stiff people and those who are always tired.

Give cooling herbs to hot people—who change to summer clothes when most others still complain of cold—or to rosy-cheeked people with iron digestions or high blood pressure.

Give moistening herbs to dry people, who drink a glass of water and pee out a glass of water ten minutes later. Such people need mucilaginous plants, which bind moisture, such as plantain (Plantago) seed, mallows, chia seed, and the like.

Dry mucous membranes need moistening. Give mallow, plantain (Plantago), or bur-marigold(Bidens) tea daily until dryness and itchiness are gone.

Dry eyes can indicate a fat deficiency.

Add healthy fats to your diet—naturally liquid or naturally hard fats. Fish oil can also be useful. Butter, lard (from organically raised animals), and coconut fat are healthy naturally hard fats. Cold-pressed oils are naturally liquid fats.

Avoid artificially hardened (hydro-genated) fats.

A fat deficiency can also show as dry, flaky, itchy skin. If this is the case, include more fats in the diet. Using oils and salves externally treats a symptom, not its cause.

To assist in fat digestion, add spices to your food and take bitter herbs 20-30 minutes before each meal. Eating a salad of bitter greens such as dandelion leaf, arugula, and endive before a meal also helps.

Warming and heating herbs help liquify mucous membrane secretions. This helps with congestive problems, such as phlegm-y coughs and sinusitis.

Secretions that flow don't get stuck, making it easier to cough and blow your nose productively.

A sock stuffed with half a chopped-up fresh onion tucked in with a child with a cold can prevent mucus accumulating in the respiratory tract. The child breathes better and the whole family sleeps easier.

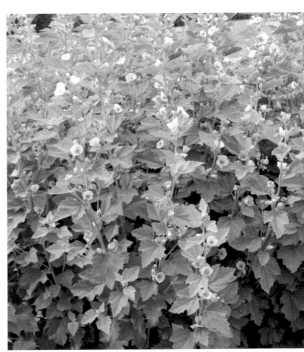

Marshmallow (Althaea officinalis) moistens.

Warming plants used internally or applied topically help warm cold extremities. On cold winter days, for example, it's lovely to sip a hot spicy tea or to massage an infused ginger or mustard oil into cold feet.

And you can reduce digestive discomfort (pain, gas, and bloating) just by adding aromatic (that is, warming) herbs to your food. Prevent the problem by taking bitter herbs 20–30 minutes before meals. Although these plants are cooling, the bitter flavor on the tongue stimulates digestive secretions.

If the digestive problems have been long-standing, it's a good idea to drink a tea made from mucilaginous (cooling and moistening) herbs, which helps heal damaged mucous membranes.

Mucilaginous and juicy cooling, moistening herbs are excellent soothers of red, inflamed eczema. Use them for small burns and itchy insect bites. Mucilaginous herbs also help treat dry or hot coughs.

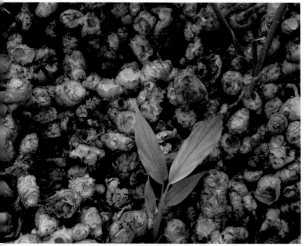

Ginger (Zingiber officinale) is warming.

Give bitter cooling herbs to those who sweat a lot. A sage tea, drunk cold, is one of our best remedies for hot flushes, but other bitter herbs are cooling, as well.

Bitter herbs can help with nausea, too, especially in "hot" people (who might gag at the very thought of ginger, a hot herb).

A dash of lemon juice or cider vinegar (sour cooling liquids) in your water bottle refreshes on hot summer days. Add a bowl of fresh berries (our local berries are almost all sour) and you're soon revived and ready to take on the world again.

A lemon–juice compress helps lower a high fever, if removing excess clothing and swapping the duvet for a topsheet doesn't help. Note, however, that elevating temperature is the body's way of fighting disease. A fever as such isn't a bad thing.

Hot flu tea with ginger or garlic

   1–2 tablespoons finely minced ginger
      or garlic
   1 teaspoon lemon juice
   1 teaspoon organic honey
   1 cup (250 ml) boiling water

Mix. Drink. This unstuffs a stuffy nose, if not with the first cup, then certainly by the second one.

Lemon–juice compress

   juice of 1 lemon
   2 cups (500 ml) cool (not cold!) water
   towels

Mix the liquids. Dip two small towels in the liquid, wring out the excess water, and apply them to the calves. Wrap with dry towels. Renew the compresses when they've warmed up.

PROBLEMS

MENSTRUAL PROBLEMS

Painful menses are all too common, especially considering how easily they can be remedied.

It's also relatively easy to prevent most PMS and heavy or irregular menses.

Treating menstrual pain due to endometriosis can be challenging, however.

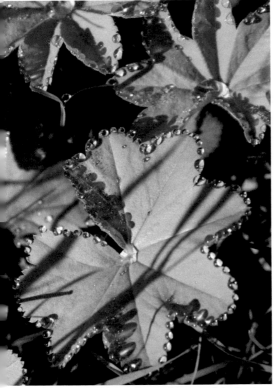

Lady's mantle (Alchemilla spp.) is one of the best herbs for women.

FEMALE HORMONES

The production of sex hormones starts in the brain. The hypothalamus produces gonadotropin-releasing hormone (GnRH), which stimulates the pituitary to produce follicle-stimulating hormone (FSH) and luteinizing hormone (LH), the principal two principal gonadotropins in humans.

FSH stimulates follicles in the ovaries to produce estrogen. The strongest follicle will become this month's egg. When estrogen reaches a threshold, the egg is released. This is ovulation.

The remaining part of the follicle—the "egg cup," as it were—is the corpus luteum. LH stimulates the corpus luteum to produce progesterone.

Important parts of our complex endocrine system, sex hormones don't function in isolation from the body's other hormones. Stress can and will affect your sex hormone levels.

Thyroid problems also can impact your menstrual cycle and its hormones.

It's always a good idea to address the liver if you have menstrual problems. A healthy liver effectively filters bits of used-up hormones from the blood.

Our bodies require building blocks to manufacture the various hormones. If we become deficient in these materials, we suffer.

14

HORMONAL NUTRIENTS

If you have hormonal difficulties, first ensure that you have the raw materials you need to produce hormones in the first place. Once you're sure of your minerals and vitamins, check your lifestyle. Herbs can help support you while you address your problem's underlying causes. If issues persist, consult your doctor.

Many menstrual problems disappear once the body receives enough magnesium, vitamin B (menstrual pain), and other nutrients (PMS, heavy or irregular menses). Use these long-term:

- Magnesium: 1200-1500 mg a day. If have painful menses and can't resist chocolate, you're magnesium deficient.
  Homemade magnesium vinegar or epsom salt baths are inexpensive and effective treatments. You'll need vitamin B, as well, to absorb magnesium.
- B-vitamins: Make sure you get 50-60 mg each of vitamins B2, B5 and B6 every day, plus smaller amounts of the other B-vitamins. (Beer yeast doesn't contain all that much vitamin B.) Magnesium is required to absorb the B-vitamins.
- Zinc: 15-30 mg a day. Sunflower seeds, sesame seeds, and almonds are good sources of zinc.
- Iron: Stinging nettle (Urtica dioica) contains plenty of iron.
- Vitamin C: Eat a large handful of your local berries every day.
- Chromium: Chromium is found in liver. If you prefer dietary supplements, take 200 µg a day. (If you can't resist sweets, you have a chromium deficiency.)

- Vitamin D: Take vitamin D capsules on those days when it's impossible to expose at least some skin to the sun for 20-30 minutes.
  D-vitamin requires calcium and fat to be absorbed. If you take vitamin D as a supplement, it's also a good idea to take magnesium and vitamin A to curb excessive of calcium absorption.
- Calcium: Foods high in calcium include dark green vegetables; nuts such as almonds, hazelnuts, and Brazil nuts; and sesame seeds. Calcium requires vitamin D to be absorbed efficiently. Also eat plenty of greens and other foods high in vitamin A.
- Protein: Add two eggs (or equivalent in whole protein) to your breakfast. Avoid soy protein.
- Fat: Eat only naturally liquid or naturally hard fats, preferably organic and (for plant-derived fats) cold-pressed.
- Multivitamin: Take a good multivitamin to ensure you get all the various dietary co-factors and trace elements.

A deficiency of B vitamins or a diet high in simple carbohydrates can cause the body to become deficient in magnesium. Its tell-tale symptoms are muscle cramps, painful menses, PMS, a craving for chocolate, and depression. Some people also get migraines or smelly sweat.

Stress, artificial hormones (for example, the pill and hormonal IUS), GERD medication, and proton pump inhibitors can create a deficiency of B vitamins. Telltale symptoms of vitamin B deficiency include hot feet, depression, mental problems, arrhythmias, and fungal issues.

The following magnesium preparations are in order of preference. The vinegar is most, the oil least desirable:

Magnesium vinegar

1 part Milk of Magnesia (magnesium hydroxIde)
4 parts apple cider vinegar

Mix. Set aside to clear for about 5 minutes. Take a tablespoonful morning and night.

If this gives you get diarrhea, you're taking too much. Lower your dose.

Magnesium vinegar can aggravate heartburn. (For more on heartburn, see page 79.)

Epsom salt (magnesium sulphate)

Add 2 cups (400 ml) Epsom salt to a warm bath. Relax and soak 15–20 minutes.

For a footbath, add ½cup (100 ml) Epsom salt to a basin of warm water. Soak your feet 10–20 minutes.

Magnesium oil

1 part magnesium chloride
1–2 parts spring water

Boil water. Add magnesium chloride and stir to dissolve. Let cool.

Massage this into your skin or apply it as a mist using a spray bottle.

If this mix irritates your skin, dilute it with water. You can also add some of this liquid to baths or footbaths.

Dosage will vary by individual. Start with a small daily amount and use a little more every day. If symptoms of magnesium deficiency don't subside, use more. If you get diarrhea, use less.

NUTRIENT-DENSEHERBS

Herbs such as raspberry leaf, lady's mantle leaf, stinging nettle, oat straw, chickweed, and red clover are high in minerals and trace elements. Make them into teas or overnight infusions. Some can be incorporated into meals as wild greens, as well.

A mineral-rich herbal tea

1 ounce (30 g) dried herb
1 quart (1 l) water

Pour water into a pan, bring to a boil. Add the herb, cover, and steep overnight.

In cold weather, bring to a boil, strain, and drink.

In hot weather, strain and drink.

Try adding honey, spices, and/or milk to your tea before you drink it.

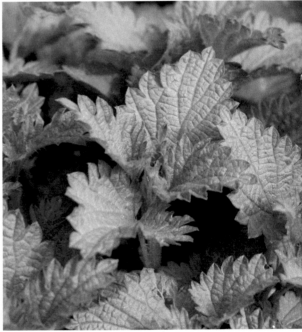

Stinging nettle (Urtica dioica) is rich in nutrients.

HELP THE LIVER

A well-functioning liver will filter parts of used hormones from the bloodstream.

If the liver is less efficient, some of these hormone parts will remain unprocessed. In this case, the blood will carry more used hormones than normal, and the hypothalamus and pituitary will secrete less stimulating hormones than normal. Thus, the menstrual cycle suffers.

An overworked liver can be due to digestive problems, such as a sensitivity to a common food. If you're sensitive to, say, dairy products or gluten-containing grains, the blood that moves from your intestines to your liver will contain more wastes than it should. Removing the offending food(s) from the diet solves the problem. If a total removal of a suspected intolerance-causing food doesn't work, you can continue to eat it: it's not a good idea to restrict your diet unnecessarily.

A lot of plants help support the liver. Try, for instance, the roots or leaves of dandelion, chicory, or burdock; the green parts of bur-marigold(Bidens spp.); the flowering tops of common toadflax (Linaria vulgaris) or turtlehead (Chelone spp.); or the roots of yellow dock (Rumex crispus), barberry (Berberis spp.), or Oregon grape (Mahonia spp..

Your liver will thank you, and your menstrual problems will diminish.

Liver tea

½ teaspoon dried dandelion root or leaf
½ teaspoon dried yellow dock root
1 cup (250 ml) boiling water

Pour boiling water over the herb, steep for 10 minutes, and strain.

Drink up to 3 cups a day.

PAINFUL MENSES

Menstrual pain usually indicates magnesium deficiency.

You don't have to think you'll die for two days every month. You don't have to skip work (or school) to lie wrapped up in a warm blanket, and you don't have to curl up in a corner hoping for the pain to end.

The pain stops right away if you chew on a piece of recently dried root of angelica or calamus.

You can also make compresses or poultices from various aromatic mint-family plants.

But although herbs can help lessen the symptom (pain), you should also address the cause: take magnesium and B-vitamins. (For more details about these nutrients, see page 15.)

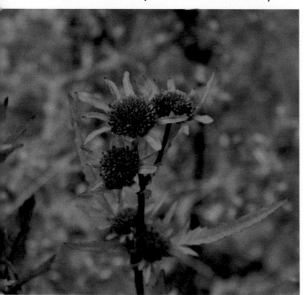
Bur-marigold(Bidens radiata) helps the liver.

ENDOMETRIOSIS

Truly bad menstrual pain can be due to endometriosis, a condition where endometrial tissue (uterine lining) grows outside the womb. This tissue responds to hormone levels: estrogen makes it grow, and a drop in progesterone makes it bleed, as endometrial tissue in the womb does.

The more cramped the area where this tissue forms, the greater the pain. Endometrial cells that grow in the Fallopian tubes can create pain intense enough to cause fainting. Chewing angelica or calamus root will lessen the pain.

Endometrial tissue in the abdominal cavity can cause scar tissue adhesions that prevent abdominal organs from sliding effortlessly against each other. You hurt when you bend this way or when you reach that way.

Castor oil packs help eliminate such internal scar tissue.

Endometrial tissue in the lungs can manifest as bloody coughing—or even pneumothorax.

If you suffer from endometriosis, you also should consider avoiding dairy products and gluten-containing grains for at least a month. The gluten-free part should start with acquiring your own cutting board (no stray breadcrumbs from others' food). Eliminating dairy should be likewise total—no cheese, yogurt, butter, milk, or any other dairy products.

If either dietary change helps reduce or eliminate your symptoms, continue with it. If you experience no change in your menstrual pain, however, go back to eating a normal, varied diet.

Suppressed memories of childhood sexual abuse can amplify or aggravate the pain of endometriosis. If you suspect this is the case, consult a good counselor. Use herbs that foster courage and compassion, such as rose, cinquefoil, or hawthorn.

Castor oil compress

1-2 tablespoons castor oil
a small cloth
hot water and a towel
 or a hot water bottle

Spread castor oil on a cloth and apply it to your lower abdomen. Warm the area with a hot water bottle or hot towel. Keep this in place for about 30 minutes.

Repeat daily.

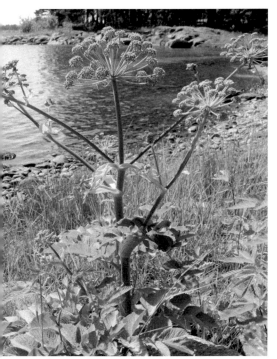

Angelica root helps with painful menses.

18

PMS

If you suffer from irritability before each onset of menses and sincerely want to get rid of your PMS, help your liver. You'll quickly notice a difference.

You should also take nutritional supplements your body needs to manufacture hormones—not only sex hormones, but all the hormones we need to feel happy.

If you really need an excuse to "clear the air," buy some shoes a size or two too small. Wear them for a day, and you'll be sufficiently irritated to explode at minor annoyances—and you'll know why.

HEAVY MENSES

Heavy menstrual bleeding can be a problem that feeds itself: anemia causes the bleeding that causes anemia. Take care of the anemia: eat iron-rich foods (including stinging nettle) regularly.

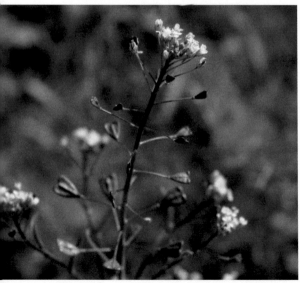

Shepherd's purse (Capsella bursa-pastoris) stops bleeding.

If that's not enough, drink iron-rich herb juices from the health food store. You'll absorb the iron in these juices more efficiently than the iron from pills, and they won't upset your stomach. They don't necessarily taste good, though. Buy a small bottle at first, and then buy more if you like its taste.

Another cause for heavy menses is too much prolactin in the blood. This can be due to dopamine deficiency. You need the same nutrients to make dopamine as you do for other hormones. (Read more about these nutrients on page 15.)

Visit your doctor if you suspect you have too much prolactin.

Herbs that curb bleeding include shepherd's purse (Capsella bursa-pastoris), yarrow, chili pepper, and cinquefoil. Take them as a tea or a tincture or eat them in your food. Repeat every ten minutes, until the bleeding stops.

IRREGULAR MENSES

If you've been taking artificial hormones such as the pill for years, your menses are likely to be irregular for a while after you stop. Your body needs time to start producing hormones on its own again. It's like removing a cast from a leg: it will take a while to rebuild those muscles and walk normally.

Help your body find its rhythm by supporting your liver and making sure your diet includes the nutrients you need to produce hormones.

If your menses are irregular and the problem isn't artificial hormones, your doctor can help you determine the cause.

POST-PARTUMDEPRESSION

The depression some mothers experience after (or before) giving birth can be due to a combination of factors.

During pregnancy, the little one "skims the cream" off the nutrients her moms diet supplies. This is as it should be: your baby needs trace elements, vitamins, and minerals to grow properly.

If the blood lost during childbirth is not soon replaced, anemia will acount for some of a new mother's tiredness.

The labor might have been draining, and the body must repair and heal damaged tissues.

A breastfed baby continues to receive nutrients from Mom to get the best start in life.

A new baby's needs can disrupt a new mother's sleep, which also saps strength.

So the growing baby receives nutrients from Mom during pregnancy and breastfeeding, Mom's body must replace lost blood and repair damaged tissues, and finally Mom must endure the strain of disrupted sleep: producing feel-good hormones under these circumstances alone poses a challenge.

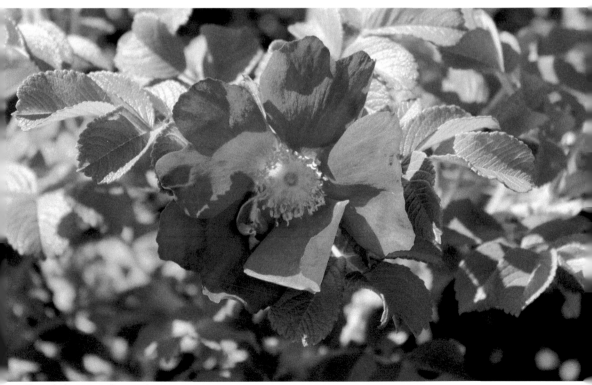

Rose helps avert depression.

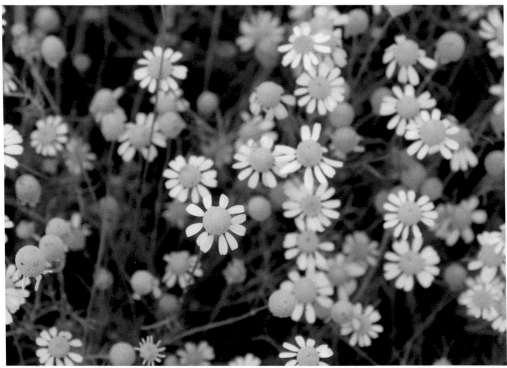

Fragrant chamomile soothes and removes cravings for attention.

And consider that life after childbirth isn't the rosy picture painted by ladies' magazines.

You still face the same housework you did before the baby arrived.

But life with baby also includes that first smile, first laugh, first steps, and first words.

Here are some tips which help you fully enjoy this time:

- Take vitamins, trace elements and minerals for at least as long as you breastfeed and/or are sleep-deprived.

- Preparing your own nutritious meals can be difficult with a little one who wants to be held all the time, so use a baby carrier or sling to keep your hands free.

- Don't worry about the dust bunnies. They're not dangerous and won't breed all that fast.

- When friends and relations ask to come admire your little one, tell them what you'd like to eat. And expect them to make the coffee and wash the dishes.

- Take relaxing herbs: milky oats tincture (Avena sativa, A. fatua) is top-notch, but so are motherwort (Leonurus cardiaca) and chamomile (Matricaria recutita). It's a good idea to give chamomile to the other family members, as well. It soothes those cravings for attention. Chamomile feels like a hug from mom.

INFERTILITY

For infertility, I recommend herbs, nutrients, dietary and lifestyle changes, and sometimes a little psychology.

You'll find a list of essential nutrients on page 15. These components are important for three reasons:

- They soothe and regulate hormone production, which makes it easier to conceive.
- They help maintain a pregnancy, lowering the risk for a miscarriage.

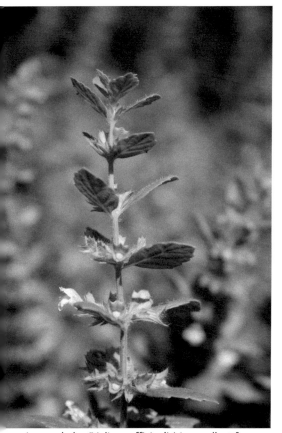

Lemon balm (Melissa officinalis) is excellent for stress.

- They help prevent many birth defects: B-vitamins (especially folic acid) lower the risk for spina bifida by 70 percent, for instance. Nutritional supplements lower the risk for cleft palate 80 percent and birth defects overall by about 60 percent.

Include enough fat, protein, and colorful vegetables. Reduce your intake of simple carbohydrates such as bread, rice, and potatoes. Because soy upsets hormone balance, avoid all processed soy products (soy milk, soy protein, soy yogurt, and so on).

Change your lifestyle to lower stress. Your body won't prepare to make a child if it's always fleeing bears and tigers.

Use calming and nervine herbs such as milky oats, rose, or lemon balm (Melissa officinalis). Cinquefoils (Potentilla spp.) and hawthorn (Crataegus spp.) can help you to assert yourself.

A menstrual cycle is essential if you want to conceive. A passionate woman athlete doesn't necessarily menstruate. She should lighten up on her training at least until she conceives.

Heavily over- or underweight women also will find it difficult to become pregnant.

Artificial hormones, as well, play havoc with our natural ones. Let your body recover from them for a few months before you try to get pregnant.

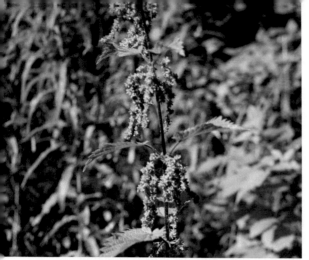

Nettle seed ready for harvest.

Some psychology might be needed when everything looks all right, and there's still no pregnancy.

One woman might try too hard. Another may harbor secret fears about what having a child will do to her life.

Fixating on ovulation is unnecessary, and making sex into a chore is outright detrimental. Research shows that women are fertile for at least nine days after ovulation, not just four or five.

Relax. Drink a little wine, nibble on some chocolate, pamper your spouse, and forget the pressure. Stress-free sex helps foster conception.

Fear of the lifestyle changes parenthood may bring likewise can interfere with conception. Promise yourself you'll hire a babysitter at regular intervals to allow for some "you" time. Once you eliminate worry, a pregnancy becomes more likely.

Herbs that promote fertility include red raspberry leaf, lady's mantle, nettle seed, carrot flower and seed, lily flower, and herbs that support the liver.

(Read about liver herbs on page 17.)

RED RASPBERRY LEAF (RUBUS IDAEUS)

Raspberry leaf is high in minerals and trace elements and strengthens female reproductive organs.

Drink red raspberry leaf tea when you want to become pregnant, stop drinking it for the first three months of pregnancy, and then resume consumption until childbirth and beyond.

Drinking the tea in the first three months of pregnancy may result in breakthrough bleeding. This isn't dangerous, but it may alarm a pregnant woman.

LADY'S MANTLE (ALCHEMILLA VULGARIS)

Lady's mantle also has a long history of strengthening women's pelvic organs. Lady's mantle also contains a lot of minerals and trace elements, and is safe to use throughout pregnancy.

Raspberry or lady's mantle tea

1–2 teaspoons dried or fresh leaf
1 cup (250 ml) boiling water

Pour boiling water over the herb, steep 5–10 minutes, and strain. Drink 2 or 3 cups a day.

NETTLE SEED (URTICA DIOICA)

Nettle seed strengthens the adrenals and the kidneys and helps maintain a calm, rested state.

The usual recommended dosage is a teaspoon of the dried seed taken every day. If you're very sensitive, however, a pinch may be enough, and if you're more robust, you might need a tablespoonful, or a teaspoon of fresh seed. Fresh nettle seed makes some people restless, while calming others.

CARROT FLOWER AND SEED (DAUCUS CAROTA)

The flowering or seeding top of carrot (or wild carrot, queen Anne's lace) works as a contraceptive, provided it's taken three times at 12-hour intervals after intercourse.

The problem with using it as a contraceptive regularly for a few weeks or months is, if you forget to take it even once, you're pregnant! (I've exploited this very characteristic to treat infertility problems.)

Because wild carrot isn't "wild" in Finland, and I can't fit very many flowering carrots in my garden, I usually tincture the flowering tops or the green or brown seeding tops. Eating ripe seeds works, too, but make sure they're organically grown.

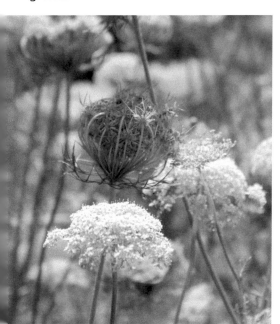
Carrot flower and a "nest" of green seeds.

Carrot flower and seed tincture

> 4 ounces (100 g) fresh flowers or seed balls of carrot
> 8 fluid ounces (200 ml) 190 proof grain alcohol (95%)

Put the herb into a glass jar, cover with the alcohol, and close the lid tightly. Steep for 2 to 4 weeks. Strain, bottle, and label (example: "Carrot flower and seed, 1:2 95%, 08.2021, Back yard").

Doasge is 15–30 drops, one to three times a day.

Take it throughout the month of your cycle, stopping for 6 days or so before you ovulate.

Carrot seeds

> ½ teaspoon dry ripe carrot seeds

Take once a day, except for your fertile time of month.

LILY FLOWER (LILIUM SPP.)

Because lily flower helps treat some kinds of cysts, I used it for that purpose with several clients. One of them promptly got pregnant, so I've used it to treat infertility ever since.

Any lily will do, as long as it's botanically a species of Lilium. I've used the petals of all true lilies in my garden, among them martagon or Turk's cap lily (L. martagon), tiger lily, Madonna lily (L. candidum), and various gorgeous lily hybrids.

I tincture the fresh petals in the same proportions as in the foregoing formula for carrot flower or seed. Dosage is two to five drops, one to three times a day.

HEMORRHOIDS

Hemorrhoids have a number of possible causes. The most common is a congested local blood supply that creates local varicosities that are more or less uncomfortable or painful.

If your movements are limited to the distance between the couch and the fridge, your blood can't really circulate in the vein around the anus. Walking for half an hour a day works wonders. Time your walk for midday, and you might also get relief from insomnia. Good herbal teas astringe the tissues of a couch potato; that is, they tighten lax mucous membranes.

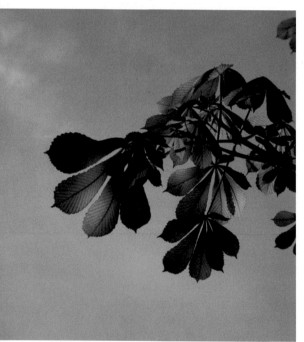

Salve made from horse chestnut (Aesculus hippocastanum) is an excellent topical treatment for hemorrhoids, varicose veins, and bags under the eyes.

Astringent herbs include raspberry leaf, lady's mantle, cinquefoil, and alder cones (Alnus spp.).

For hemorrhoids that develop due to something bearing down on the vein around the anus, relief will depend on the pressure's source: If it's a saddle or bicycle seat, go for a walk every now and then. If it's a growing baby, walks can help, but they won't be enough.

Use these herbs alone or together in tea, bath, sitz bath, or compress: chamomile, yarrow, ground ivy (Glechoma hederacea), catnip, mallow, and mullein.

Salves also can help enhance local blood flow. Make a salve from yarrow, horse chestnut, and/or catnip, and apply it after each bowel movement. And insert a suitably sized wedge of fresh potato now and then.

Food sensitivity also plays a role in the development of some hemorrhoids. Determine which food offends and remove it from your diet.

Use the aforementioned plants and support your liver with herbs such as dandelion, burdock leaf, yellow dock root, and barberry root.

Few people are cursed with "athlete's" hemorrhoids, which arise when muscles are so tuned they push part of the mucous membrane out the rectum. They find relief in teas of relaxing herbs such as catnip, chamomile, and valerian.

MIGRAINE

A typical migraine headache affects one hemisphere of the brain with intense, pulsing, debilitating pain lasting from two hours to as long as 72.

Some simple causes of migraine include the following.

- Magnesium deficiency. Approximately four out of five migraine sufferers are found to be magnesium deficient. Excessive consumption of sugar and simple carbohydrates (bread, sweets, rice, potato, fresh juice) draw on magnesium reserves.
In addition, our over-farmed soils are depleted of minerals such as magnesium. Commercial fertilizers contain a only few major nutrients—and magnesium isn't one of them.

- Vitamin B deficiency. Our bodies need B vitamins in order to absorb magnesium. Stress draws on our vitamin B reserves. The cycle is most starkly demonstrated in schoolchildren who experience migraine before important exams: Stress depletes key B-vitamins. This prevents the body from absorbing magnesium. Lack of sufficient magnesium then causes a migraine.

- Aspartame, monosodium glutamate, and/or benzoate sensitivity. One out of 10 migraine sufferers can trace the onset of their headache to consumption of these additives.

- Tyramine sensitivity. One in 20 suffers gets a migraine from eating foods rich in tyramine, such as chocolate, soft cheeses, and red wine.

- Few people are outright allergic to a given food. When a client tells me, "I always get a migraine when I eat [this food]," I can only reply, "You should avoid [that food], then."

- Ubiquinone (coenzyme Q10) deficiency. In this case, taking supplemental CoQ10 for a few weeks takes care of the problem.

Overwhelmingly, though, magnesium deficiency is the root cause of most chronic migraine. Refer to page 16 to learn how to make magnesium vinegar and epsom salt baths, and remember to take your B vitamins.

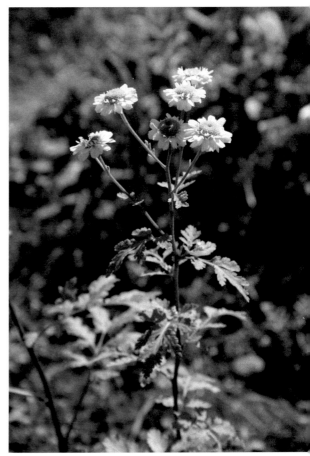

Feverfew (Tanacetum parthenium) can help with symptoms of migraine, but it's more important to address the root cause.

26

DIGESTIVE PROBLEMS

The two most common causes for digestive upset are underactive digestion and food sensitivity.

UNDERACTIVE DIGESTION

If you seem to react to a new food every month, or if you belch constantly, you probably suffer from underactive digestion.

The list of foods that cause you lower gut pain, a woozy feeling, and/or bloating gets longer and longer. You wonder whether soon you'll be unable to eat anything.

But of course you will. Do this:

- Eat only warm foods. If you must eat ice cream, for example, eat it warm. Warm even your salads before you eat them.
- Avoid sugar. Take chromium supplements and add protein to your breakfast to diminish your sugar cravings.
- Avoid drinking beverages with meals. These slow your digestion. If you must drink sodas or energy drinks, take them warm.
- Avoid alcohol altogether.
- Reduce your coffee intake. If you really can't give it up, add warming spices to your cup, such as cardamom or cinnamon.
- Add warm or hot spices to all your food. Also take digestive bitters or bitter herbs 20–30 minutes before each meal. You'll find short lists of aromatic and bitter plants on pages 8 and 9.

Take these steps and in just a few weeks you'll notice an improvement in your digestion.

Once your digestion regularly works as it should, you can try a cold salad now and then, or take a very occasional glass of wine.

Just remember that if you return to your old habits, your digestion soon will be underactive again.

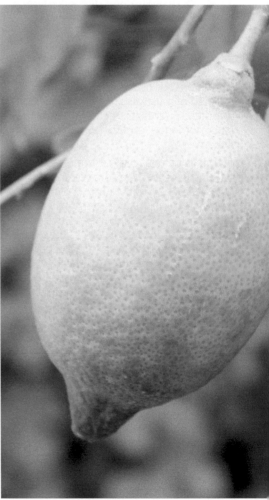

Citrus peel is aromatic and bitter.

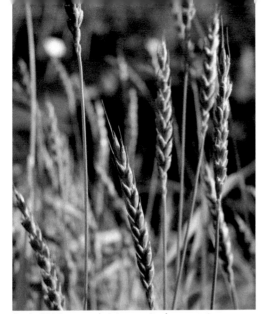

Spelt (Triticum spelta) is a grain that contains gluten.

FOOD INTOLERANCE

Food intolerance lies at the root of a variety of problems.

If nothing seems to help your constipation, for example, you're probably eating a food you're sensitive or allergic to.

If you alternate between diarrhea and constipation, consider possible food sensitivities.

If eating a certain food always causes gut cramps, excessive belching, or serious flatulence, an allergy or sensitivity to it probably is the cause.

Common food intolerances include gluten-containing grains (wheat, spelt, rye, barley, and oats) and dairy products. But everyone's different. Solanaceous plants (potato, tomato, bell pepper, cayenne or chili pepper, eggplant, tomatillo, to name a few), citrus fruit, eggs, onions, and food additives (glutamate, aspartame, benzoate, artificial coloring, and the like) all can trigger allergic reactions and sensitivities.

If you're having trouble pinpointing the cause of your digestive reactions, try eliminating the one food you can't imagine ever going without.

Or keep a food diary. On the left side of an open notebook write down everything you put into your mouth and the time you did so. Include even toothpaste, mouthwash, and lipstick. On the right side, note how you feel at various times of the day. After two weeks, you may notice a pattern.

Unfortunately, skin-prick allergy tests are not always reliable. But if you thoroughly remove a suspected food or food group from your diet for two weeks, and then go back to eating normally, returning symptoms will tell you what you need to know.

Once you know what you're reacting to, you must eliminate the culprit completely from your diet. If you react strongly to wheat, for example, your gut will react for 10 days to a single cookie. If you must do without dairy, learn to drink your morning tea or coffee black without that splash of milk. Instead, try adding lemon to your tea, or coconut milk to your coffee.

Going just two weeks completely without gluten or solanaceous plants can prove to you just how widely food sensitivity symptoms can range

One may be sensitive to wheat or other gluten-containing grains without having celiac disease as such. Those intolerant of lactose (milk sugar) may react to milk proteins, as well. And sensitivity to solanaceous plants can manifest as joint pain rather than digestive upset.

SMALL WOUNDS AND BRUISES

In summer, herbs to treat wounds and bruises can be found growing just about everywhere.

Crush or chew a plantain (Plantago spp.) leaf to bring some juice to its surface, and then apply the leaf to a small wound or bruise. Fix it in place with an adhesive bandage, if you like. Plantain grows almost everywhere, and all Plantago species work.

Calendula brings vivid color to a garden, and it's great for wounds. Apply fresh petals or use dried whole flowers or petals.

St. John's wort (Hypericum perforatum and related red-coloring species) is excellent for wounds and helps treat the swelling of sprains and bruises. Flowering St. John's wort plants are easy to find growing in dry summer meadows. Simply gather a few fresh flowers or flower buds, crush them to release the plant juices (No other yellow flower turns blood-red when you crush it), and apply them to your ouchie.

Make oils or a salves from these herbs to use outside the flowering season (see page 7). Oils and salves made from calendula and plantain can be made from either dried or fresh plant parts, but anything made from St. John's wort requires fresh flowering tops.

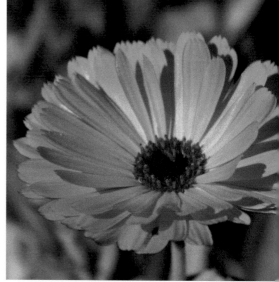

Calendula is a beautiful wound-healing herb..

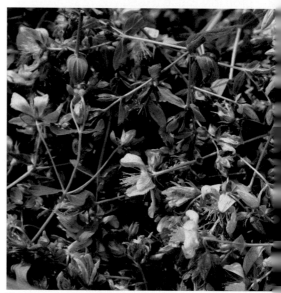

The flowering tops of St. John's wort.

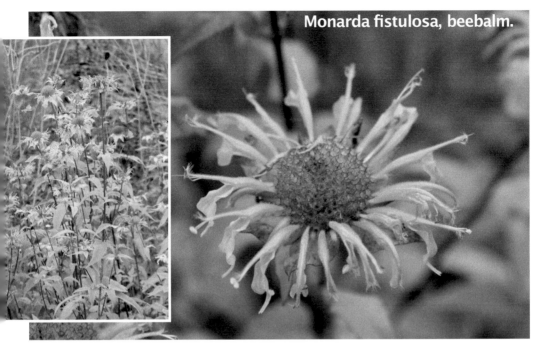

Monarda fistulosa, beebalm.

BEEBALMS

Lovely spots of color in the garden and fiery medicinal plants.

Monarda species: Also called horsemint and bergamot, as

- scarlet beebalm, oswego tea (Monarda didyma), also called fragrant balm, crimson beebalm, scarlet monarda
- lemon beebalm (Monarda citriodora), also called lemon mint, purple horsemInt
- wild bergamot (Monarda fistulosa), also called horse-mint

among other species. Fiery oregano species such as Greek oregano (Origanum heracleoticum) and hot thymes can be used in the same ways.

Taste: Hot, aromatic.

Energetics: warming, drying.

Family: Mint family, Lamiaceae.

Annual or perennial: Harvest from summer to fall.

Habitat and cultivation: Beebalms are North American plants. I've seen southern species grow in sand, but those species that survive northern winters thrive in moister and more fertile soil.

Beebalms like sun or half-sun.

Because beebalms hybridize so readily, it's best to buy perennial species from nurseries so you can be reasonably sure you'll get what's on the label. This is less certain with seeds.

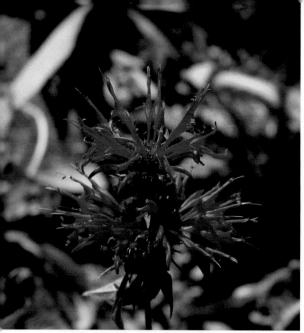

The flower of scarlet beebalm (Monarda didyma 'Cambridge Scarlet').

Flowers of annuals such as lemon beebalm (Monarda citriodora) will vary in color, but I find it a nice surprise—"Ooh, such a deep purple!"; "Wow! Now that's pink!"—and, of course, every shade between.

Sow seed indoors in March or April, and transfer the tiny plants outdoors in late May or early June.

Appearance: Beebalms have showy colorful flower heads. The flower of scarlet beebalm is bright red and that of wild bergamot is pink. Most perennials available at commercial nurseries are hybrids.

Although other beebalms blossom in tall, successive whorls, lemon beebalm's flowers are particularly showy. The spikes can top 3 feet (a meter), and the plants will continue blossoming at the top until frost kills them. (I'm not sure why lemon beebalm is called that. I have yet to come across one with a lemony taste or scent.)

Look-alikes: Beebalms can resemble catnips, mints, or nettles, before they flower.

Important constituents: Beebalms contain essential oils, the most important constituents of which are thymol and carvacrol. These are the main constituents in the essential oils of fiery thymes and oreganos as well.

PICKING AND PROCESSING

The flower head is the fieriest part of the plant. The uppermost leaves are quite hot, as well. The flower itself—the most colorful part of the flower head—can be exceedingly tasty, quite aromatic, and even anise-y.

Pick the flowering tops of perennial beebalms as long as they look healthy—once or twice from mid–July to mid–August.

Cut the flowering tops of annual beebalms in autumn before frost kills them.

Spread your harvest to dry on a bedsheet spread on a layer of newspapers, or dry them in a dehydrator, or hang them in bundles to dry in a shady spot.

Or use the fresh flowering tops to make honeys, elixirs, and tinctures.

Sometimes, it's impossible to find healthy green beebalm unaffected by white splotches of powdery mildew. (I've read that some native American groups traditionally harvest beebalm only if it is mildewed.)

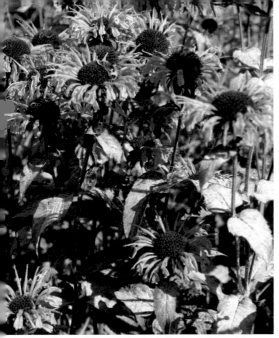

Powdery mildew on the leaf of a beebalm cultivar.

EFFECTS AND USES

Beebalms are hot, which is why they help keep airways open when we get coughs and head colds. To use, eat a fresh flower head, or drink a hot beebalm tea, and keep tissues on hand. Your nose will promptly start to drain.

Continue to drink your beebalm tea after your head cold is gone. Because it promotes local circulation, it speeds recovery.

For coughs, you can also take beebalm syrup or honey. Leave the flower heads in the liquid and eat them, too, for your warming-herb needs. The flower heads stay very fiery even stored in honey.

Use beebalms for sore throat, too.

Because of their fieriness, beebalms can be helpful for tinnitus caused by inner ear stagnation. Drink the hot tea or take the tincture regularly until the buzzing and humming stops.

Beebalms reduce nervousness. Give a beebalm tea a try when you're too tired to fall asleep.

Use beebalms for tummy aches and flatulence, and for other digestive problems. They can even help relieve diarrhea.

A hot tea of beebalm, ginger, or thyme can help relieve nausea if the sufferer is also pale and listless. If red-cheeked and vital, however, a cool peppermint tea or a dash of vinegar may be more appropriate.

Use the hot tea to bring on late menses, as well. (It won't help if menses are late due to pregnancy, though.)

The hot beebalm tea and a warm poultice or compress can help menstrual pain.

Beebalm tea

1 teaspoon dried flowering tops
 or 2 teaspoons fresh
1 cup (250 ml) boiling water

Pour boiling water over the herb, steep 10 minutes, and strain.

Sip for nausea, or drink a cup or two as needed for indigestion, flatulence, sore throat, head cold, flu, and cough.

Sweeten the tea to taste for respiratory problems, but leave it unsweetened to treat digestive issues.

Beebalm honey

fresh crushed flowering tops
 or whole flower heads
fresh organic honey

Pour honey over the herb in a glass jar, cover, and leave in a warm spot (on top of the fridge, for instance) for 2 months. Straining is optional.

Take 1-2 spoonfuls of the honey or honeyed herb for flu or cough.

32

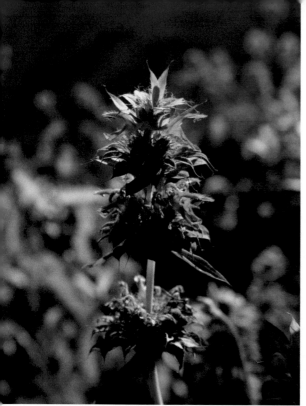

The flowering tops of lemon beebalm (Monarda citriodora).

Beebalm tincture

From fresh herb:
  4 ounces (100 g) fresh flowering tops
  8 fluid ounces (200 ml) 190 proof
    grain alcohol (95%)

From dried herb:
  4 ounces (100 g) dried flowering tops
  20 fluid ounces (500 ml) 120 proof
    grain alcohol (60%)

Put the herb in a glass jar, cover with alcohol, and close the lid tightly. Steep 2–4 weeks, strain, bottle, and label (example, fresh: "Beebalm, 1:2 95%, 8.2021, my garden"; example, dried: "Beebalm, 1:5 60%, 12.2021, Christine's herb garden").

Dosage is 5–30 drops, 1–3 times a day.

For tinnitus, take 3–10 drops, 3 times a day.

Beebalm syrup

Make a syrup from flowering tops using the recipe on page 1.

Take a spoonful of the syrup as needed for respiratory tract infections.

Beebalm compress and poultice

  1 handful dried flowering tops
    or two handfuls fresh 1 quart (1 l) water

Pour boiling water over the herb, steep 15 minutes, strain, and let cool until just skin-comfortable.

Compress: Dip a cloth in the tea, and squeeze out excess liquid. Put the moist, hot cloth on the belly and leave it there 30–40 minutes.

Poultice: Fold 1–4 tablespoons hot, moist herb into a square of cloth. Keep the poultice on the belly 30–40 minutes.

A poultice stays hot for a bit longer than a compress.

FOOD USES

Use the colorful parts of the flowers (the petals) to decorate summery salads, cakes, and drinks.

The flowers of wild bergamot taste of anise, and those of scarlet beebalm are almost like candy. Taste the others before using them to determine what note you may be adding to your foods.

Use small amounts of the fiery parts as you would oregano and marjoram.

WARNINGS

Avoid beebalms if you're pregnant or nursing.

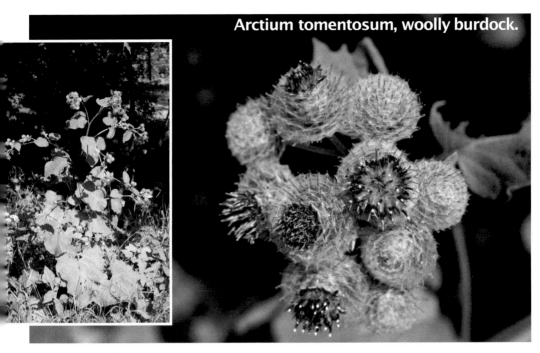

Arctium tomentosum, woolly burdock.

BURDOCK

It strengthens the appetite and digestion, makes you pee, and is a great wild food.

Arctium species: Including
- greater burdock (Arctium lappa), also called beggar's buttons, gobo
- lesser burdock (Arctium minus), also called button–burand burweed
- woolly burdock (Arctium tomentosum), also called downy burdock

among other species. Burdocks hybridize readily.

Taste: The leaf is bitter. The root is mild and a little nutty.

Energetics: The leaf is drying and cooling. The root and seeds are drying and moistening.

Family: Daisy family, Asteraceae.

Biennial: Dig the roots the autumn after their first summer. Pick the leaf in summer. Harvest the seeds the fall after the plants' second summer.

Habitat: Burdocks love gravelly, permeable soil. They are found in ditches, meadows, along roadsides, and in fields.

Cultivation: You can grow burdock in rows, much like carrots. Plant the seeds in fall or early spring. Give the plants plenty of room: a single burdock plant grown in fertile soil can fill a 3–foot square (1 m^2).

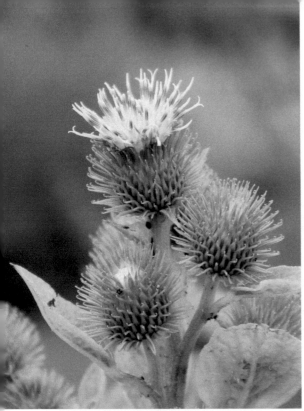
Lesser burdock (Arctium minus).

Gobo is an Asian cultivar of greater burdock. Its roots are used like other root vegetables, in soups and stews. Wild burdock roots can be used the same way.

Appearance: In its first summer, burdock will sprout only a lowish leaf rosette.

The next summer, it will send up a flower stalk that can be as tall as 8 feet (200 cm). The flower stalk has a few leaves, but most of the leaf mass grows lower down, below 2 feet (60 cm).

The large taproot goes straight down.

Burdock is perhaps easiest to recognize from its large hooked burrs (flower buds, flowers, and seed heads) that readily attach themselves to clothing and animal fur. Burdock has no sharp spines.

The leaves are rhubarb-like and large, but bitter. The leaf stems are hollow.

Look-alikes: Before it flowers, it's easy to confuse burdock with both types of coltsfoot (Tussilago farfara and species of Petasites) and with rhubarb (Rheum rhabarbarum).

Coltsfeet lack taproots, and they flower before they grow leaves. The fuzz on upper side of Tussilago leaf is easily rubbed off, revealing a smooth surface.

Petasites plants grow enormous single leaves. In late summer, they can become as large as umbrellas.

The tops of rhubarb leaves aren't fuzzy, and their leaf stems are not hollow.

The flowers resemble those of thistles. Thistles have sharp spines, where burdocks only have hooked flower heads.

Important constituents: The root is rich in vitamins (among others, A, B1, B2, B3, and C) and minerals (as calcium, potassium, iron, magnesium, zinc, and selenium), but note that minerals will be present in any herb only if they are first present in the soil the plants grew in.

If a soil is low in selenium, for example, eating a burdock grown in it won't help remedy your selenium deficiency.

By fall, the root will contain 20–50% inulin, which is a sugar we can't metabolize and not the hormone insulin. The root also contains 5–12% mucilage, some bitters, proteins, plant acids, and flavonoids.

The seed contains 15–30% oil, bitter substances, plant acids, and vitamins A and B2.

The leaf contains bitter substances and flavonoids.

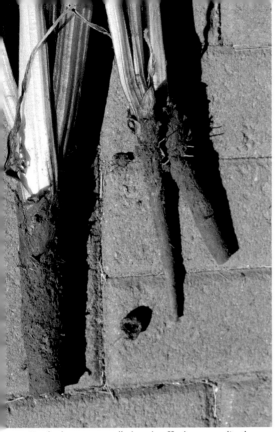

Burdock roots usually break off when you dig them up.

Leaf

It's easiest to gather burdock leaf from where a lot of burdock grows, rather than from just a single plant here and there. Pick a leaf or two from each healthy plant, and your basket will fill in no time.

For quality dried leaf, follow this procedure:

1. First, cut the larger leaf veins crossways every inch (2-3 cm) or so. Otherwise the leaf will dry poorly, with only the edges turning burdock leaf's normal blue-green and the inner leaf area turning first yellow-green, then brown, and finally black.

2. Next, suspend your leaves from a string to dry. If you choose to spread them flat instead, you must arrange them to prevent overlapping. Because the leaves go utterly limp as they dry, overlapped leaves will fuse into a solid mat that quickly becomes moldy.

PICKING AND PROCESSING

Root

Dig the root before the plant flowers, in fall or spring. The root beneath flowering plants is woody, as it must anchor the heavy flower stalk. After the plant has flowered, the root is dying.

Burdock likes gravelly soil, so you're unlikely to get very far down with a shovel before the root breaks off. It's normal to get only 5-7 inches (15-20 cm) of a burdock root. A good digging stick may yield longer burdock roots.

Wash the roots (leaving the root bark intact) and cut them into quarter-inch (5 mm) slices. Spread the slices to dry, or tincture them.

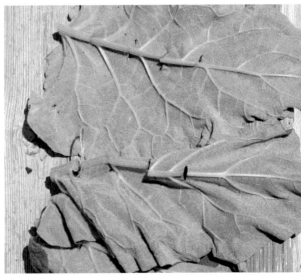

To dry burdock leaf successfully, first cut the larger leaf veins.

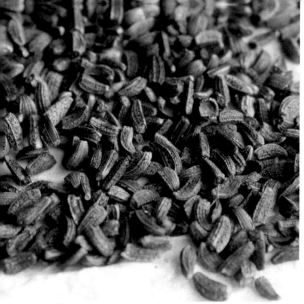

Clean burdock seed.

Seeds

Picking the seeds is happy work. A good burdock stand will fill a large basket in 10 minutes.

Processing your seed harvest is anything but fun, though, as the seeds are surrounded by itchy hairs and the seed heads' hooks will stick to everything.

Gather yellow-gray branches in seed on a dry day and cut off the seed balls. Put them in a tallish bucket—preferably outdoors—get a baseball bat (or wooden potato masher), and use it to pound the mass in the bucket.

Don sturdy garden gloves, place a sieve over a bowl, and pour the now-compacted material into the sieve. Rub the mass against the sieve: most of the itchy hairs will accumulate in the bowl. Discard the hairs under a bush or somewhere out of the way of bare feet.

Grasp handfuls of material and, holding it slightly above your pounding bucket, massage it between your two gloved hands. The seeds will fall into the bucket.

When you see no more seeds in your burdock mass, deposit this debris, too, under the aforementioned bush.

Now fill the bucket with water and stir vigorously. The heavy seeds will sink and the fluff will float. Pour the floating debris under the same lucky bush.

Repeat until no more fluff comes to the surface.

Finally, drain the seeds in your sieve, and then spread them to dry.

This really is the most efficient way to get clean burdock seed.

The seeds will harbor a few insect larvae, but because the pounding evicted them, they're now visible. Do remove them.

Use the seeds in tinctures, or crush and dry them to use in teas or capsules.

EFFECTS AND USES

Root

Burdock root is nutritious. It enhances fat digestion and strengthens the body's blood-purifying organs—namely, liver and kidneys.

The root can be very effective against longstanding skin problems such as psoriasis, atopic eczema, and acne. You'll notice improvement within a few weeks of regular use. Continue taking burdock regularly even after those first few weeks, if the problem diminishes or even clears up.

Burdock root helps deliver fat to dry, fat-starved skin.

Because the root helps strengthen the kidneys, it's useful for gout and related joint pains.

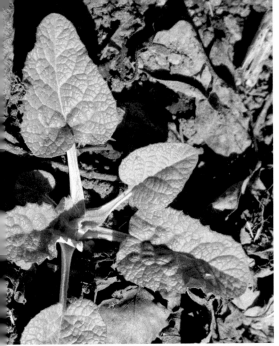

A burdock leaf rosette in early spring. Dig up such rosettes to get at burdock roots. The larger the leaves, the larger the root.

Burdock root is diuretic (it makes you pee more than usual). If you have low blood pressure, burdock root can so reduce your fluid levels (and therefore, your blood pressure) you may grow dizzy or even faint. People with low blood pressure should take burdock and such diuretics with salt, which helps the kidneys hold onto water. Because the root contains potassium, its diuretic effect won't contribute to a potassium deficiency.

I think burdock root tastes sweet and a little nutty, but it does have a slight bitterness to it. The bitter taste enhances appetite and digestion.

The root contains large amounts of inulin, a sugar. Although we can't metabolize inulin as such, our large intestine's beneficial bacteria love it, and so burdock root helps treat some digestive problems.

Some people with irritable bowel syndrome (IBS) or similar severe gut upset, however, might do well to avoid all such inulin-rich starchy roots.

Burdock root is mildly laxative, as it makes for softer stools.

Burdock root is one of the herbal ingredients in the tea blend Essiac, which is used to help treat various cancers. Try the root as a tea or, if you can take it, as a tincture, to supplement other cancer treatments.

Burdock root tea or tincture helps with minor uterine prolapse. Start taking burdock root as soon as possible after the prolapse. Take a few drops of the tincture every hour or two, or sip the tea continuously during the day, until the connective tissue has strengthened enough to keep the uterus in place.

Give burdock root a try in rectal prolapse, as well.

Burdock root helps reduce premenstrual tension (PMS) in women prone to it, probably because burdock strengthens the liver and the kidneys. (Fierce premenstrual mood swings can also be due to too much stress).

For PMS, also supplement your diet with the nutrients you need to balance hormones (see page 15). Excessive stress and severe hormonal upsets deplete at least vitamin B and magnesium, but take other nutrients, as well.

Externally, rub an infused oil of burdock root or leaf into your scalp if you suffer from abnormal balding (alopecia). (Read more about alopecia on page 43).

Leaf

Because of its bitterness, burdock leaf stimulates both appetite and digestion.

The leaf is also strongly diuretic. If your urine is dark and possibly burning, this is the herb for you: drink burdock leaf tea regularly. (Because the leaf contains potassium, its diuretic activity won't deplete your potassium reserves.)

The leaf is helpful externally for skin problems such as eczemas, sunburn, bruises, and abrasions. Use an infused burdock leaf oil or a salve made from the infused oil, or use the leaf in poultices or compresses.

Apply burdock leaf poultices to bedsores and cold sores (fever blisters, herpes simplex), and try the leaf both externally and internally for shingles (herpes zoster).

A bain-marie with burdock leaf and oil.

Rub the fresh leaf to release some of its juice and apply it to insect bites. Relief!

Try a burdock leaf tea for cracked, dry heels and for dry skin elsewhere.

Add a little chopped burdock leaf to some egg white and apply the mix to minor burns.

Apply crushed or blanched burdock leaf to draw pus to the surface to drain and heal an abscess.

For dandruff, use the leaf both internally and externally.

Try burdock leaf for Dupuytren's contracture (palmar fibromatosis), an inherited connective tissue disorder that gradually draws the fingers toward the palm. Little to nothing short of surgery treats this problem effectively, so burdock leaf is worth at least a try. Apply the crushed fresh leaf to the hands, or rub an oil or salve made from the leaf onto the shortened tendon.

Use the root internally and the leaf externally for some joint problems and gout, and for long-term skin problems such as psoriasis and atopy. For psoriasis, also take vitamin D and try a gluten-free diet. For atopy, it's a good idea to go completely dairy-and/or gluten-free.

Apply vinegared burdock leaf to scrapes, abrasions, and bruises, and to swellings from trauma.

Seed

Use the seeds to treat the same issues you'd use the root for. The seeds work quickly, alleviating symptoms fairly fast. The root works more slowly, but by helping both liver and kidneys it address "root" causes.

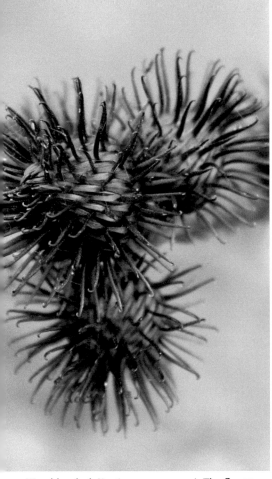

Wood burdock (Arctium nemorosum). The flower bud is about to open.

Burdock seed is diuretic and greasy. It helps with long-term skin problems, and because it helps bring the proper amount of fat to the skin, it's good for dry skin, as well. Try burdock seed (or root) internally if your heels are always cracked and dry, or if your skin is always too greasy.

The seeds help some kidney and bladder stones. Take a tincture especially if you have mucilage in your always dark urine, or if your dark urine included sand.

Burdock root decoction

1-2 teaspoons dried root
1 cup (250 ml) boiling water

Add root and water to a pan, bring to a boil, continue to boil 20 minutes, and strain. Drink 1-3 cups a day for at least 2 weeks.

Burdock tea

1-2 teaspoons dried or fresh leaf or seed
1 cup (250 ml) boiling water

Pour boiling water over the herb, steep 5-10 minutes, strain. Drink 2-3 cups a day.

Burdock oil and salve

Make an oil from fresh or dried leaf and make a salve from that (see recipe, page 7).

Burdock tincture

From fresh herb:
4 ounces (100 g) fresh burdock root, leaf, or seed
8 fluid ounces (200 ml) 190 proof grain alcohol (95%)

From dried herb:
4 ounces (100 g) dried burdock root, leaf, or seed
20 fluid ounces (500 ml) 120 proof grain alcohol (60%)

Put the herb in a glass jar, cover with alcohol, and close the lid tightly. Steep 2-4 weeks, strain, and bottle. Label (example, fresh: "Burdock root, 1:2 95%, 5.2021, behind the barn"; example, dried: "Burdock seed, 1:5 60%, 12.2021, by the compost heap").

Dosage of tinctured root is 30-90 drops, 3 times a day.

Dosage of leaf or seed tincture is 10-25 drops, 3 times a day.

Burdock leaf compress and poultice

1-2 fresh or dried leaves
1 quart (1 l) water

Pour boiling water over the herb, steep 15 minutes, strain, and cool to just skin-comfortable.

Compress: Dip a cloth in the tea, and squeeze out excess liquid. Put the moist, hot cloth on the skin that needs soothing and leave it there 30-40 minutes.

Poultice: Fold 1-4 tablespoons hot moist herb into a square of cloth and leave the poultice on the affected area 30-40 minutes.

A poultice stays hot for a bit longer than a compress.

LadyB's vinegared burdock leaf

1-2 fresh burdock leaves
organic apple cider vinegar

Cut burdock leaves lengthwise into inch-wide ribbons, and then roll them up. Put the rolls into a glass jar and cover with vinegar. If the lid is metal, first covering the top of the jar with plastic wrap and closing the lid over that will prevent corrosion.

Unroll and apply the vinegared leaf to bruises, scrapes, abrasions, and similar minor ouchies.

FOOD USES

Flower stalk

The inner, white part of burdock flower stalk, before the flower buds have fully developed, is very tasty. Slice off the stalks at ground level, remove the leaves (save them separately), and peel the stalk.

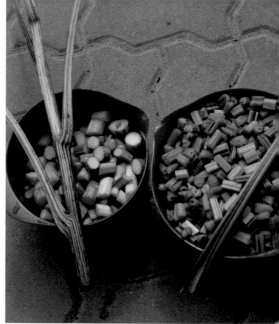

Burdock flower stalk and leaf stalks, sliced and ready to boil.

Cut the peeled white part of the stalk into half-inch (1-2 cm) segments. (The few greenish fibers left on the peeled parts may be faintly bitter.)

If the inner stalk is hard to cut, no amount of boiling will make it softer. Discard this particular flower stalk, and look for softer ones.

The upper part of a burdock flower stalk can be soft and tasty even when the buds are turning into flowers, but by then the flower stalk itself is becoming bitter.

Boil the whites of the flower stalks with salt and serve with a dash of butter or a good sauce. If your taste buds tell you that this is bitter, add something sour, such as lemon juice or vinegar.

Use the reserved leaves in medicine.

Leaf stalk

The leaf stalk is a good enough wild green; I don't find it bitter. It's fibrous, so this, too, is best sliced into half-inch (1-2 cm) pieces. Boil in salted water and add the pieces to stews and soups, or serve with a dash of butter and some lemon juice.

Root

Burdock roots are a great wild food. Wash (no need to peel), slice, and boil them, and then serve them with a good sauce.

Digging the roots is hard work. It's far easier to cultivate the root ("gobo") and harvest the homegrown roots from your soft garden soil.

Fried burdock root

Cut the washed roots into quarter-inch (5 mm) slices. Fry in fat or oil, and add a little soy sauce.

If you find the roots bitter, soak the slices in cold water for 15 minutes before frying.

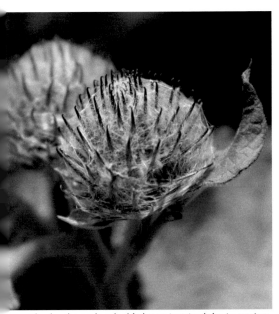

The hooks on burdock's burrs inspired the invention of Velcro. The hooks are clearly visible in this closeup of a flower bud.

OTHER USES

Velcro mimics the hooks of burdock's burrs. Mischievous children (and childish adults) often toss the burrs onto each others' sweaters, or arrange them on their own to write their names.

The not-quite-that-childish can form wreaths from the flowering burrs.

Assemble the burrs into artful sculptures: no need for glue, and you can detach and rearrange them.

Give your hair some shine with burdock leaf:

Burdock leaf hair rinse

2 ounces (50 g) fresh burdock leaf
1 quart (1 l) boiling water

Pour boiling water over the shredded leaf, steep 5-10 minutes, strain.

Let cool. Use as your final hair rinse for a few weeks.

WARNINGS

It's a good idea to avoid taking burdock in early pregnancy. Use it only in the last trimester, if your ankles are very swollen.

The burrs' hooks will cause a very unpleasant inflammation if they get into the eye, so handle the plant with care.

Although the leaf used externally can cause contact dermatitis in sensitive people, this reaction is very rare.

The hairs around the seeds inside the burrs are extremely itchy.

Burdock leaf is strongly diuretic, as are the seeds and roots. If you have low blood pressure and wish to use burdock, remember to increase your salt intake.

BALDNESS OR ALOPECIA

You can do a lot for some types of involuntary baldness.

Try to find the reasons for your baldness, and do something about them:

- The cause for full-body baldness can be found in the diet. Completely removing gluten-containing foods from your diet can be enough to reverse full-body baldness.
- Alopecia areata (spot baldness) can signal too much stress. Take potentilla or agrimony to give you the oomph to remove your stressors, and take lemon balm, hawthorn, and/or milky oats to help your nerves.
- Thinning hair, on the head or elsewhere, especially in menopausal women, can indicate an underactive thyroid. Try a gluten-free diet and avoid other simple carbohydrates. And get a thyroid test.

- Male pattern baldness is a sign of too much testosterone. Testosterone thickens the skin of the scalp, which ultimately starves the hair follicles. You can try herbs that inhibit testosterone production, such as saw palmetto(Serenoa repens) or peppermint, but then you might grow breasts as a side effect.

General herbs that help stimulate hair growth include stinging nettle, burdock, and horsetail. Use them in teas and hair washes.

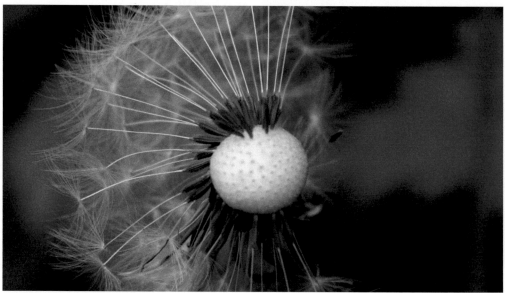

An almost bald dandelion puff.

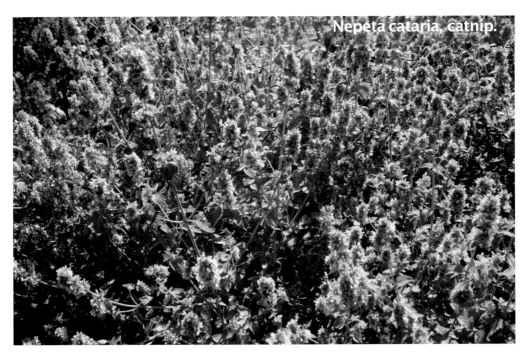
Nepeta cataria, catnip.

CATNIP

A relaxing plant that drives cats wild.

Nepeta cataria: also called catmint, catnip.

Other useful Nepeta species include:

- Lemon catnip (Nepeta cataria 'Citriodora')
- Faassen's catnip, garden catmint (Nepeta ×faassenll)
- Caucasus catmint (Nepeta grandiflora)
- Siberian catnip (Nepeta sibirica, Dracocephalum sibiricum), also called Siberian catmint
- Dwarf catnip (Nepeta racemosa), also called dwarf catmint, Persian catnip

Taste: Aromatic, almost hot. The scent is, in fact, a smell.

The scent and taste of lemon catnip are refreshingly citrus.

Other catnips are mildly aromatic, missing the "bite" of true catnip. Their scent, too, is disagreeable.

Energetics: Heating or warming, drying.

Family: Mint family, Lamiaceae.

Perennial: Harvest from summer to fall.

Cultivation: Catnip is easy to grow from seed. It likes a sunny spot in porous soil and will freely self-seed. Catnips and catmints do not propagate by root runners.

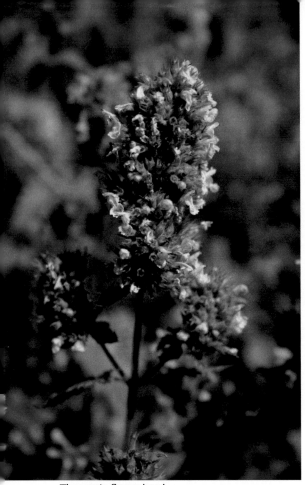

The catnip flower head.

Your neighborhood cats may shred a newly planted true catnip plant, so use seed when you can.

Cats show far less interest in other catnip and catmint species.

Because it's a hybrid, Faassen's catnip won't grow true from seeds. Propagate it by root division, instead.

Catnip and Caucasus catnip seedlings both have bluish stems when grown in sunny spots, so don't pull up all your Caucasus catnip seedlings! Taste the leaf: if it has a bite, it is, in fact, true catnip, not Caucasus catnip. (Caucasus catnip once strove to take over my garden, and in pulling it, I eradicated my true catnip, as well.)

Leave seedlings that have a lemony scent, too (unless you're overrun by lemon catnip).

Appearance: Like all mint family plants, catnips have opposite leaves and square stems. The leaves resemble stinging nettle leaves, but they're soft (and don't sting!).

Catnip flowers are white with small pink dots and grow in spikes.

Flowers of other catnip species range in color from light to dark purple.

Catnip and Caucasus catnip are usually less than a yard (1 m) tall.

Siberian catnip, which tops 5 feet (1½ meters), won't stay upright in my garden. Instead, it falls over and covers smaller plants.

Dwarf catnip and Faassen's catnip are low-growing plants often used as ground covers.

Catnips have that telltale smell of cat urine. The scent of lemon catnip is a refreshing exception.

Look-alikes: Catnips resemble stinging nettles before they flower. There are similar plants in the mint family, as well, but few have the smell of catnips.

Important constituents: Catnip is nutrient-dense. Provided these elements abound in the soil where it grows, it can contain magnesium, manganese, iron, calcium, potassium, and selenium.

Other constituents include essential oils (carvacrol, nepetol, thymol, geraniol, pulegone), tannins, and bitter substances.

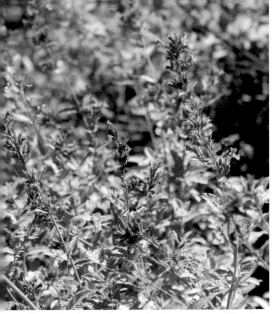
Flowering Caucasian catnip (Nepeta grandiflora).

PICKING AND PROCESSING

Cut catnip in full flower just above the lowest healthy leaf pair, or pick the flowering tops.

Take half the plant now and the other half in a few weeks' time, or coppice a stem here and another there.

Any catnip is useful, but I prefer true catnip (Nepeta cataria)—and, of course, lemon catnip.

Dry your harvest in a shady, well-ventilated spot, in hanging bundles or spread on a cloth. Or dry it in a dehydrator below 95 °F (35 °C). When all stems break instead of bending, the herb is really dry. Strip the dry leaves from the stems.

Store your dried catnip in airtight glass jars.

Or tincture fresh catnip.

Use catnippy true mints as you would catnip. Corn mint (Mentha arvensis) and water mint (Mentha aquatica) have a strong, catnippy smell.

EFFECTS AND USES

Catnip is calming, diaphoretic (makes you sweat), antispasmodic (helps with menstrual and digestive cramps), mildly emmenagogic (bringing on menses), and mildly narcotic (makes you sleep).

Calming: Use a tea or tincture of catnip when you're nervous, restless, or sleepless. It won't touch serious sleeplessness or restlessness, but it's reliable for mild nervous problems. It lessens stress and helps you relax when you go to sleep.

Also take catnip for stress-caused digestive upset, headaches, or irritability.

Catnip will help if you suffer from nightmares.

Catnip is suitable for infants. Breastfeeding moms can take catnip to deliver it in their milk, or baby can sip spoonfuls of lukewarm tea.

Fever and colds: Use catnip for fevers and colds in adults and children.

Hot catnip tea, or tincture taken in hot water, help if the fever brings on sweating, headaches, irritation, or a sore throat. Take hot catnip to open stuffy noses and sinuses.

The tea is especially good for the dotted diseases of childhood. It calms and brings on sleep.

Try the hot tea for bronchitis, as well.

Combine it with yarrow and hot blackcurrant or elderberry juice.

Digestive problems: Use catnip as a warm tea or warm compress for mild gut or menstrual cramps and gas. If the gut problems are due to nerves, catnip is excellent.

Give catnip tea to a child with diarrhea.

If your baby is colicky, give cooled catnip tea (or try chamomile or fennel teas).

Because catnip is somewhat bitter, it strengthens digestion. The bitterness is most pronounced in cooled catnip tea.

Menstrual problems: Take magnesium and B vitamins if you have both menstrual cramps and cravings for chocolate.

If you have menstrual pain and a nervous disposition, take some catnip.

(Note: catnip may increase menstrual flow a little.)

Catnip can help bring on menses if you don't bleed when it's your time of month (secondary amenorrhea).

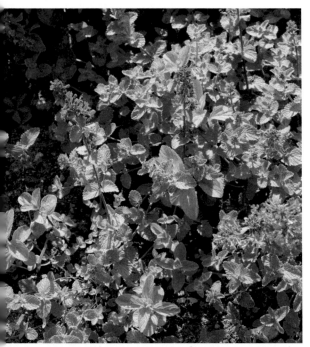

Faassen's catnip (Nepeta ×faassenii) is a ground cover.

For menstrual problems, catnip prepared as juice pressed from fresh flowering tops is strongest. Also try catnip tea combined with warm catnip compresses.

Catnip may be so effective for menstrual problems because it's mineral-rich.

Toothache: When your little one is cutting teeth, catnip can alleviate her discomfort. Dip a clean cloth in cooled catnip tea, put it in the freezer, and then give the frozen cloth to your child to chew on.

Catnip helps toothachey adults, as well. Chew a leaf and keep it against the achy side. Remove the leaf when the pain stops. Book time at your dentist if the pain returns!

Other: Catnip is mildly diuretic.

Because it's high in iron, it's good for anemia.

A hot compress of catnip leaf helps aches and inflammations, as well as sprains, strains, bruises, and swelling from trauma.

Try a salve made from the fresh leaves for hemorrhoids.

A foot bath calms the restless and nervous. It also moistens the skin.

A hair rinse of strong catnip tea is good for the scalp.

Juiced catnip

Use fresh-juiced flowering catnip tops right away, or freeze the juice in ice-cube trays. Move the cubes to airtight bags or cartons and label (example: "Catnip, fresh juice, 7.2021, my garden").

Take a tablespoonful 2-3 times a day.

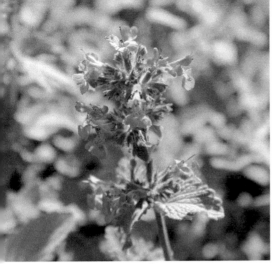

The flowerstalk of Faassen's catnip.

Catnip tea

   2 teaspoons fresh crushed catnip
      or 1 teaspoon dried catnip
   1 cup (250 ml) boiling water

Let the water cool 5 minutes (it shouldn't be boiling hot for catnip tea). Pour the hot water over the herb, steep 10 minutes, and strain. Squeeze as much liquid as you can from the herb. Drink 1–3 cups a day.

To improve the flavor, add mint (for fevers) or chamomile or fennel (for digestive problems).

Strong catnip tea

   1 ounce (30 g) dried catnip
   mint or lemon balm (optional)
   2 cups (500 ml) boiling water

Cool the water 5 minutes (it shouldn't be boiling hot for catnip tea). Pour the water over the herb, steep 10 minutes, and strain.

Take 2 tablespoons, 1–3 times a day.

Children can take 2–3 teaspoons just once or every 10 minutes to relieve painful gas.

Add thyme, chamomile, mint, or lemon balm to improve the flavor, if you like.

Catnip tincture

From fresh herb:
   4 ounces (100 g) catnip fresh flowering tops
   8 fluid ounces (200 ml) 190 proof
      grain alcohol (95%)

From dried herb:
   4 ounces (100 g) dried catnip
   20 fluid ounces (500 ml) 120 proof
      grain alcohol (60%)

Put the herb in a glass jar, cover with the alcohol, and close the lid tightly. Steep 2–4 weeks, strain, and bottle. Label (example, fresh: "Catnip, 1:2 95%, 9.2021, Grandad's garden"; example, dried: "Catnip, 1:5 60%, 12.2021, my garden").

Dosage is 10–60 drops, 1–3 times a day, or 1–3 drops as needed—before meals for digestion or before bed to calm restless.

Catnip and fennel tincture

   1 ounce (25 g) fresh catnip
   1 ounce (25 g) dried fennel seed
   vodka (80 proof, 40%)

Use four times as much vodka as you have herbs. That is, for 1 cup of herbs, use 4 cups of vodka.

Put the herb in a glass jar, cover with vodka, and close the lid tightly. Steep 2–4 weeks, strain, and bottle. Label (example: "Catnip and Fennel tincture, 9.2021").

Use ¼–½ teaspoon in a little water for digestive upset, gas and bloating or hiccups.

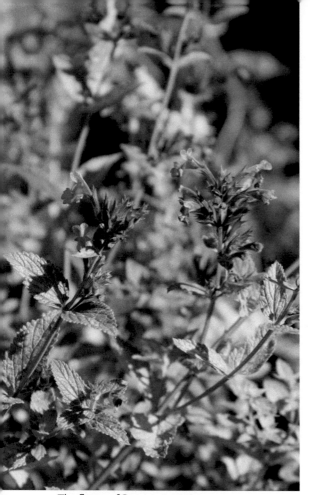

The flower of Caucasus catnip.

A catnip bath or foot bath

  2 quarts (2 l) boiling water
  dried or fresh thyme

Fresh herb: Cover herb with water.

Dried herb: Put herb in a pan and add triple the amount of water.

Bring to a boil, let simmer for 15 minutes. Strain. Pour into bathwater or a basin and add enough cold water to make for a comfortable bath. Soak–

 and enjoy, or put your feet into a foot bath for 10–20 minutes.

This is very relaxing.

Catnip oil and salve

Make an oil from fresh catnip and make salve from it (see recipe on page 7).

Catnip compress

  1 handful dried catnip
    or 2 handfuls fresh
  1 quart (1 l) water

Pour boiling water over the herb, steep 15 minutes, strain, and let cool until just skin–comfortable. Dip a cloth in the tea, and squeeze out excess liquid. Put the moist, hot towel on the hurt spot, or on the belly for menstrual pain, and leave it there 30–40 minutes.

Catnip Sleepytime bundle

  2 tablespoons dried catnip
  8–inch–square (20x20 cm) cotton cloth
  string

Put the herb in the middle of the cloth, lift the corners, and tie a catnip bundle. Keep this under your pillow.

If your housecats like catnip, use other herbs instead. If you must use catnip in a pillow bundle, use a sewing machine to really sew that bundle shut.

FOOD USES

Use lemon catnip as you would any other lemony herb—for instance, in fruit salads, or to impart a lemony flavor to a jar of water.

OTHER USES

Some cats go wild over catnip flowers. Others prefer dried valerian root. Some don't like either.

I'm told that the scent of both valerian and catnip closely resembles feline sex pheromones. That makes these plants guilty of false advertising; I haven't given them to cats for years.

If you do wish to make a catnip cat toy, though, make sure it can survive substantial biting and shredding:

Cat toy

dried or fresh catnip
5–by–10–inch(15x30cm) cloth rectangles

Fold the cloth in half the short way and sew two sides shut. Turn the pouch inside–out, fill it with catnip, and sew the last side shut.

Give one to your cat—or to a sleepless, catless friend.

WARNINGS

Because catnip can increase menstrual flow, it can increase the risk for spotting in pregnancy. Spotting isn't dangerous, but it's an unnecessary stressor. Avoid catnip if you're pregnant.

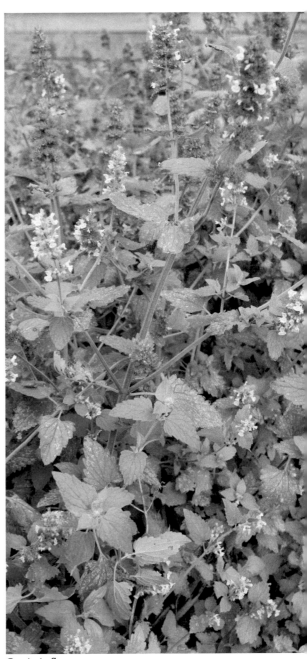

Catnip in flower.

CELERIAC AND ITS USES

Don't use celeriac if you're sensitive to it.

Celery (Apium graveolens) strengthens appetite and digestion. Both celery and celeriac or "knob celery" (Apium graveolens var. rapaceum) work. Add them to stews, soups, and other cooked foods.

Chew a few celery seeds to relieve digestive problems. They're very effective for the discomfort of overeating, nausea, and for gas and bloating.

Use the seeds for gout, as well, when you're out of "gout berries" such as strawberries, blackcurrants, and cherries.

Using celeriac to increase sex drive is common in Germany, where there's even a nursery rhyme on the theme. It probably works because it enhances pelvic blood circulation.

Of course, any libido-enhancing herb will work better, if both partners know that it works.

Celeriac salad for two

Salad:
> ½cup (150 ml) finely grated fresh celeriac or diced boiled celeriac
> 1 apple, grated
> 1–2 tablespoons crushed walnuts

Dressing:
> 3 heaping tablespoons (50 ml) mayonnaise
> 3 heaping tablespoons (50 ml) unsweetened whipped cream
> dash of lemon juice
> salt

Mix and serve.

Note: Raw celery or celeriac can irritate a sensitive stomach.

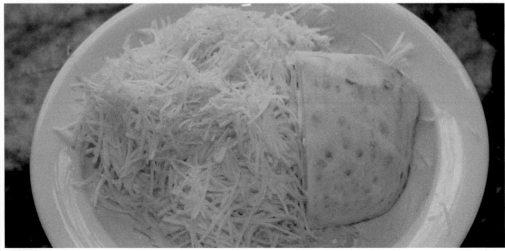

Finely grated celeriac.

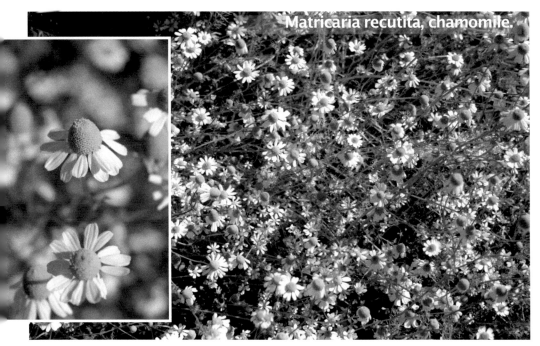

Matricaria recutita, chamomile.

CHAMOMILE

A gentle medicinal plants which removes cravings for attention.

Matricaria recutita: Also called camomile, German chamomile, scented mayweed, and sweet chamomile.

Taste: Aromatic, sweet, bitter.

Energetics: Warming, drying.

Family: Daisy family, Asteraceae.

Annual: Harvest in summer.

Its relative Roman chamomile (Chamaemelum nobile) is perennial. Harvest it, too, in summer.

Habitat: Chamomile is a declining native in Finland. Pineapple weed (Matricaria matricarioides), which can be used like chamomile, is an alien species on the increase here.

Both thrive in sunny spots in poor but well-drained soil. Look for them along sunny roadsides or on gravel and sand.

Pineapple weed is perhaps easiest to notice on a rainy day, when the scent of trampled plants is strongest.

Cultivation: Sow seeds in fall or spring in a sunny spot. Don't cover the seeds.

In rich soil you get a lot of leaf and very little flower.

Chamomile seeds remain viable for only about a year.

Chamomile thrives along the edges of the potato patch. It hasn't grown well in my herb garden.

Appearance: Chamomile is delicate and only about 4–16 inches (10–40 cm) tall. Its scent and taste are mild and aromatic. Chamomile flowers are yellow with white petals. Fully open flowers are hollow inside.

Pineapple weed appears more robust. It grows to only 4–12 inches (10–30 cm), and its greenish flowers have no petals.

The leaves of both are threadlike, similar to dill leaves.

Look-alikes: Mayweed (Tripleurospermum perforatum, scentless chamomile, scentless mayweed, false chamomile) is larger than chamomile, lacks the scent, and its flowers aren't hollow.

The leaves of oxeye daisy (Leucanthemum vulgare) aren't dill-like, the leaf and flower have no scent, and the flowers aren't hollow.

Important constituents: Chamomile contains essential oils (chamazulene, alpha-bisabolol), flavone glycosides, coumarins, salicylic acid, and mucilage.

PICKING AND PROCESSING

Herb books often say to pick only the flowers, but I suggest doing this only if you're harvesting the flowers to sell. You can, of course, pick the flowers one-by-one, but it's faster to get a good grip on the stem of the flowering plant and cut the flowers straight into your basket.

Try using a berry picker: the flowers will separate easily from their stems if you wait until afternoon when the ground is dry, and the roots retain their grip on the earth.

I prefer to cut the flowering plants to one or two hands' height above the ground,

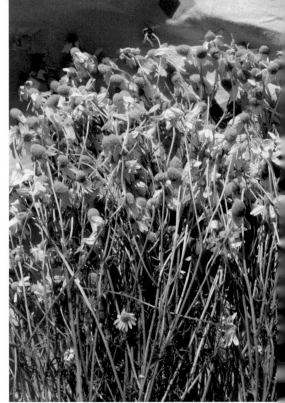
Flowering chamomile drying on a piece of bedsheet.

because the green parts work, as well. Of course, the leaves and stems aren't quite as strong as the flowers.

Pull plants with their roots from overcrowded stands. Remove the roots and any yellow or brown leaves.

Dry chamomile whole or cut into inch-long (2–3 cm) pieces.

The yellow part of the flower is chamomile's strongest part.

Spread chamomile to dry on a layer of newspaper or an old bed sheet.

Or use a dehydrator set lower than 86 °F (30 °C), with the flowers on a piece of lightweight cloth.

If you hang chamomile in bundles, the flowery parts will fall off as they dry. Encase the bundles in a paper bag ventilated with large holes.

EFFECTS AND USES

Use pineapple weed (Matricaria matricarioides) as you would chamomile.

Roman chamomile (Chamaemelum nobile or Anthemis nobilis) is a bit more bitter than chamomile. This makes it more effective for liver and digestive problems.

Chamomile removes cravings for attention. You won't do outrageous things just to get noticed if you first take some chamomile. Perhaps that's why chamomile is so good for those who complain without suffering. (Use cinquefoil instead, if you suffer without complaining.)

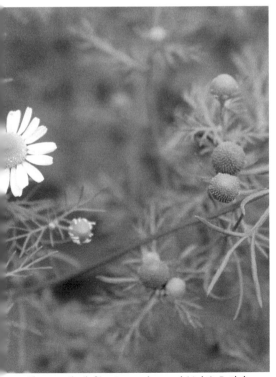

Chamomile (left), pineapple weed (right). Both have dill-like leaves.

If your child kvetches, and neither food nor sleep help, try some chamomile. It can stand in for Mommy's hugs when Mommy can't hug.

Chamomile tea or tincture is calming, and helps even the overtired get some sleep.

Chamomile calms the stomach, as well, resolving mild gut cramps and digestive upsets due to nervousness.

Take it for bloating, gas, and diarrhea, and when you're recovering from diarrhea, nausea, or vomiting.

Chamomile has also been used to treat peptic ulcers.

Try chamomile, if your baby suffers from colic. One mom told me that her baby always calmed down exactly 20 minutes after taking some chamomile tea. Nothing else touched the colic. (It also might be a good idea to change your diaper-changing practices: don't fold baby's legs above her; instead, learn to roll baby to either side. You'll soon get the hang of it—especially if baby stops crying her heart out for hours at a time.)

Chamomile helps with menstrual pain (but remember to take magnesium and B vitamins if your menses are painful).

For cold, flu, sinusitis, cough, sore throat, or gum disease, drink a hot chamomile tea, gargle with it, inhale the steam, or spritz a little cooled tea to the back of your throat.

For symptoms of post-traumatic stress disorder, try 3-6 cups of strong chamomile tea every day until the sufferer starts to relax and live normally again. (Engage in other therapies, as well!)

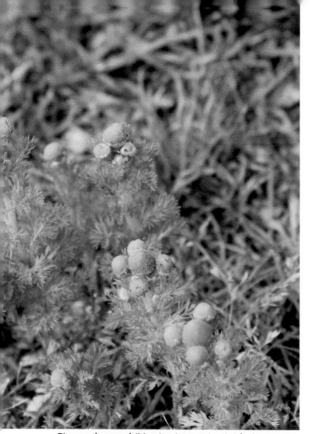

Pineapple weed (Matricaria matricarioides).

Chamomile can ease the transition away from antidepressants. Drink up to 8 cups a day for the first few days. Never stop taking psychotropic medication on your own!

Externally, chamomile treats minor skin problems, small wounds, itchy or red eczema, sunburned skin, and hemorrhoids. Regular use will even help with acne rosacea.

Chamomile is helpful for joint pain, nerve pain, and earache.

Use chamomile for acne: steam the pimply skin with a hot chamomile tea, or use lukewarm chamomile compresses.

Make an infused oil from chamomile and use it for massage, or as a relaxing, moisturizing oil.

A chamomile bath relaxes, helps relieve inflammations and itchy skin, and accelerates the healing of wounds.

Use chamomile tea bags, a few drops of tincture in boiled cooled water, or tea in compresses for mild eye problems. (Never touch the side of a compress that will touch the eye. Your eye doesn't need more problems.)

As a rinse for blonde hair, use a strong chamomile tea. (Strain it well, or you'll be brushing flower parts from your hair for a week!)

A hot chamomile pack is a mild and effective treatment for aches and pains. Use it for earache, as well.

Chamomile tea

1-2 teaspoons dried or fresh chamomile
1 cup (250 ml) boiling water

Pour boiling water over the herb, steep 5-10 minutes, strain.

Drink warm for digestive problems, take a cup for gas and bloating after a meal, or drink 1-3 cups a day for a few months for acne and rosacea.

Make your tea even stronger and gargle for sore throat and gingivitis.

Cool the tea to a comfortable temperature and use it as a compress or wash for skin problems, aches, and small wounds.

Chamomile tea for babies

1 teaspoon chamomile tea
½ cup (100 ml) warm water

Mix. Give a teaspoon to treat colic.

For a breastfeeding baby, mom can take the rest of the chamomile tea.

Chamomile elixir

fresh chamomile
fruit brandy or vodka
liquid organic honey

First fill a glass jar with chamomile, then fill to a third with liquid honey, and finally add brandy (or, in a pinch, vodka) to the top. Steep 2-4 weeks out of the light. Strain.

Take one or two spoonfuls for colds, cough, and flu, or when you need a hug.

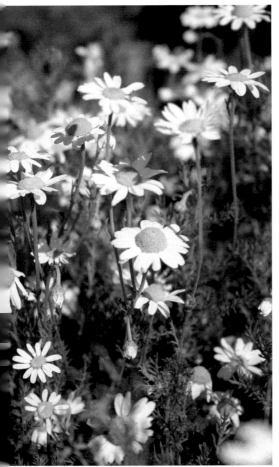

Roman chamomile (Chamaemelum nobile).

Chamomile tincture

From fresh herb:
4 ounces (100 g) fresh chamomile
8 fluid ounces (200 ml) 190 proof
grain alcohol (95%)

From dried herb:
4 ounces (100 g) dried chamomile
20 fluid ounces (500 ml) 120 proof
grain alcohol (60%)

Put the herb in a glass jar, cover with alcohol, and close the lid tightly. Steep 2-4 weeks, strain, and bottle. Label (example, fresh: "German chamomile, 1:2 95%, 7.2021,around the potato patch"; example, dried: "Pineapple weed, 1:5 60%, 5.2021,my yard").

Dosage is 15-30 drops, 3 times a day.

Chamomile compress

a handful of dried chamomile
or two handfuls of fresh chamomile
1 quart (1 l) water

Pour boiling water over the herb, steep 15 minutes, strain, and let cool until just skin-comfortable. Dip a cloth in the tea, and wring out excess liquid. Put the moist, hot cloth on the hurt spot, eczema, or itchy skin and leave it 30-40 minutes.

A chamomile bath

dried or fresh chamomile
water

Fresh: Put the herb in a 2-quart(2 l) pan and add water to cover.

Dried: Put the herb in a 2-quart(2 l) pan and add triple the amount of water.

Bring to a boil, steep 15 minutes, strain, and add to bathwater. Adjust the temperature for comfort, get in, and enjoy!

Chamomile steam inhalation

2-3 tablespoons chamomile
1 cup (250 ml) boiling water

or

1 tablespoon chamomile
1 tablespoon thyme
1 tablespoon marjoram or oregano
1 cup (250 ml) boiling water

Add the herb to a bowl, pour boiling water over it, and set the bowl on a table. Take a large towel and drape it to make a tent for your head and the bowl. Inhale the steam for 10 minutes (or three songs on the radio).

A chamomile steam helps with colds, flu, sinusitis, sore throats, and coughs.

Chamomile oil and salve

Make an oil from the fresh or dried flowers and make a salve from that (see recipe, page 7).

Use the oil or salve for skin troubles, small wounds, and aching joints.

A warm chamomile pack

4 ounces (100 g) dried chamomile
muslin bag

Fill the bag with chamomile. Heat it on the radiator or in a low oven (100-125 °F or 40-50 °C). Apply to aches and pains.

FOOD USES

Chamomile tea is a wonderfully relaxing tea to serve guests.

Or add fresh chamomile flowers or leaves to desserts.

OTHER USES

Use a lukewarm chamomile tea as a facial wash.

Use the decoction as a rinse for blonde hair.

Spray cooled, strained chamomile tea on seedlings if they're plagued by mold and fungi. You might not save those already affected, but you could well save the others.

Chamomile hair rinse

3 teaspoons dried chamomile
1 cup (250 ml) boiling water

Add the herb and water to a pan, bring to a boil, simmer 10 minutes, cool, and strain.

Use as a hair rinse.

WARNINGS

Sensitive people may react badly to chamomile. This is more likely if they also react to mugwort or yarrow. Don't use chamomile if it gives you an allergic reaction!

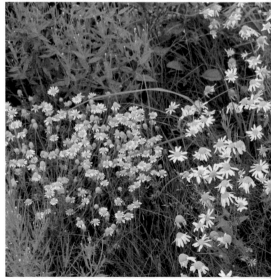

The chamomile on the left is much smaller than the scentless mayweed on the right.

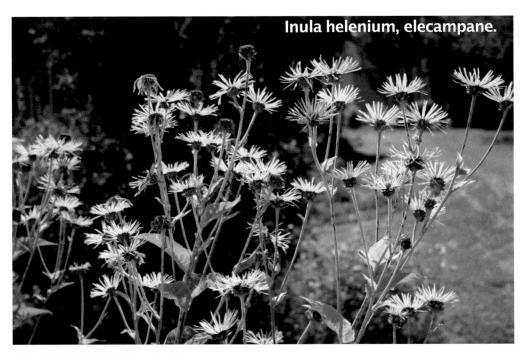

Inula helenium, elecampane.

ELECAMPANE

Good for coughs and for exhaustion.

Inula helenium: Also called elf dock, horse elder, horse-heal, scabwort, velvet dock, wild sunflower, yellow starwort.

Taste: At first aromatic, soon bitter, and then tingly.

Energetics: Warming, drying.

Family: Daisy family, Asteraceae.

Perennial: Dig the roots when the ground isn't frozen. Best when dug in fall.

Habitat and cultivation: Plant elecampane in clay or in rich soil. A mature elecampane requires about 10 square feet (1 m²). The plant and its roots will grow even larger if you feed the soil every few years.

Appearance: The flower stalk of elecampane can grow to 7 feet (2 m) tall.

The flowers are yellow with sparse petals.

Elecampane is large before flowering as well: the leaves will reach lengths of 3 feet (1 m). They are soft and slender. The underside of the leaf is grayish white.

The roots are gray-white with a red-brown bark.

Look-alikes: Young elecampane can look like dark mullein (Verbascum nigrum), but the leaf of dark mullein stinks.

Comfreys (Symphytum spp.) may be confused with elecampane when both are young. Comfrey leaves are green underneath, and rough.

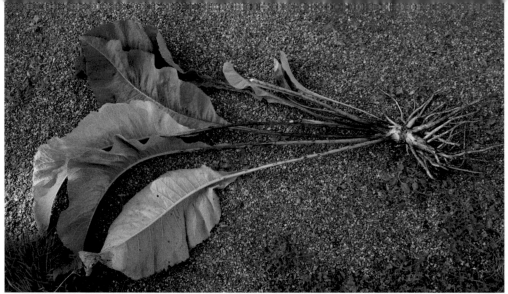

A 3-year-old elecampane. The leaves are a yard (1m) long!

Important constituents: The root contains up to 40% inulin in fall. Inulin is a sugar we can't metabolize, but which feeds friendly gut bacteria. It's not insulin, and it doesn't affect diabetes. In large amounts, inulin can cause gas and bloating.

In addition, elecampane root contains bitter substances, flavonoids, and 1-3% of essential oils.

PICKING AND PROCESSING

The fall-dug root of elecampane can be almost sweet.

During other times of year, the root is very bitter.

The taste is interesting: at first it's aromatic ("This tastes great, I wonder why it isn't used more?"), about half a minute later the bitterness hits ("Right—now I know!"), and perhaps half a minute later your mouth tingles, and continues tingling for about half an hour ("Wow, what a root!").

Dig elecampane roots from plants 3 years old or older.

By 5 years, elecampane plants will have roots the size of a human head. If you don't need quite that much, poke around the plant to find finger-thick straight side roots, instead.

If you don't have elecampane seedlings, replant the crown of a dug-up elecampane: cut stalks back to a half-inch (1 cm). Cut the roots to 2-4 inches (5-10 cm).

You can plant side roots, too, if they have buds.

Rinse the dirt, earthworms, and small stones off your roots outdoors, using a hose or a water barrel. Scrub off the remaining dirt in a basin. You don't have to remove the root bark.

Despite their huge size, elecampane roots are easy to cut. You can get nice, quarter-inch (5 mm) slices with just a bread knife. Side roots smaller than that can be split.

Spread the roots to dry, or use a dehydrator.

Try the fresh roots in syrups and tinctures.

EFFECTS AND USES

Elecampane root works well for productive, phlegmy coughs. Chew on the root, drink a tea made from it, or take some elecampane honey, syrup, or tincture. Elecampane also works as a steam inhalation.

Take elecampane root whenever the cough is due to a digestive problem. Digestive problems can cause coughs like this: when we can't properly digest proteins, we won't have raw materials for white blood cells. Without them, our immune system is weakened. If our weak spot is the respiratory tract, coughs, colds, and flus will take turns with us: as soon as one infection is over, the next one begins.

The root gives relief if the cough stems from tension or grief.

Because elecampane root is aromatic ("spicy") and bitter, it works nicely for digestive problems.

It also helps with throat irritation caused by tough, viscous mucus.

Use elecampane for phlegm-ysinusitis. (Chronic sinusitis almost always is caused by fungi or molds. A simple course of an antifungal will help. Eliminate sources of mold in your living or working environment.)

Try elecampane for leukorrhea and other excessive vaginal secretions.

And take elecampane for some urinary tract problems.

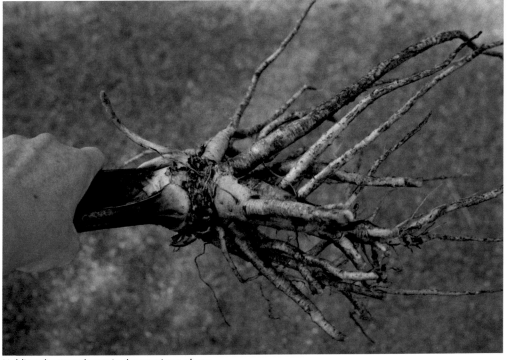

Holding the root shown in the previous photo.

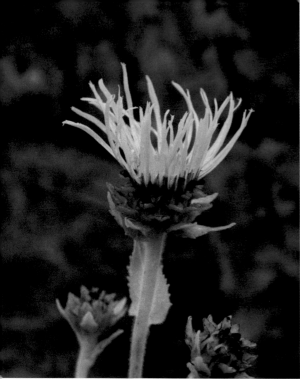

Elecampane flower.

Elecampane helps those suffering from chronic fatigue, listlessness, dreariness, weakness, and exhaustion. Try it for the exhaustion brought on by a stressful job or for the debility of old age.

Try it for Lyme disease, as well, if the symptoms include exhaustion.

In England, the use of elecampane for exhaustion goes back to ancient times, when the root was used to treat "elfshot," where strength and vitality were thought to leak away via punctures from elven arrows.

Herbalist and author Zoe Hawes explains it nicely: "Humans who wander into elven territory, dance endlessly without rest and become exhausted as a result but they can't stop dancing when the music starts up again. Inula is earthy and solid. The scent is base. The taste bitter. It grounds the feet and the mind follows".

Elecampane also can help get a handle on difficult infectious diseases, as MRSA or tuberculosis.

Elecampane tea

1-2 teaspoons dried or fresh roots
1 cup (250 ml) boiling water

Pour boiling water over the root, steep 5-10 minutes, strain.

Drink 1-3 cups a day.

Elecampane decoction

2 teaspoons dried or fresh roots
1 cup (250 ml) boiling water

Add root and water to a pan, bring to a boil, steep 12-15 minutes, and strain.

Drink 1-3 cups a day.

Elecampane maceration

1 teaspoon dried or fresh roots
1 cup (250 ml) cold water

Pour water into a pan, add the root, steep 4-12 hours. Bring to a boil, and strain.

Drink hot, 1-3 cups a day.

Christopher's decoction for the exhausted

Herb blend:
2 parts elecampane root
2 parts lovage root
1 part cinnamon
1 part licorice root

Decoction:
1-2 teaspoons of herb blend
a few crushed cardamom seeds
1 cup (250 ml) cold water

Bring herbs and water to a boil, simmer 10 minutes, cool, and strain.

Drink 3-4 cups a day for a few months.

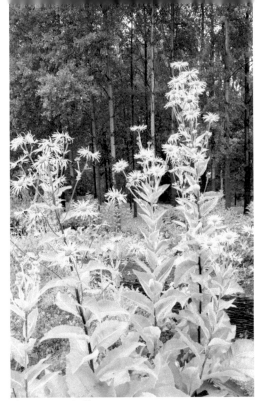

Elecampane in flower.

Elecampane steam inhalation

2-3 tablespoons dried or fresh roots
1 cup (250 ml) boiling water

In a bowl, pour boiling water over the root and drape a large towel over it to make a tent for your head. Inhale the steam for 10 minutes (or about three songs on the radio).

The steam opens the nose and sinuses and can break up congestion in the inner ear, helping some kinds of tinnitus.

Elecampane honey

Use the recipe on page 2, or make elecampane honey like this:
½cup (100 ml) dried or fresh roots
10-18 ounces (300-500 g) organic honey

Combine root and honey and steep 2-6 weeks. Remove the root matter and take a spoonful as needed.

Elecampane syrup

Make a syrup using the recipe on page 1.
Take a spoonful of syrup as needed.

Elecampane tincture

From fresh root:
4 ounces (100 g) fresh root, sliced
8 fluid ounces (200 ml) 190 proof
grain alcohol (95%)

From dried root:
4 ounces (100 g) dried root, sliced
20 fluid ounces (500 ml) 120 proof
grain alcohol (60%)

Cover the roots with alcohol in a glass jar, and close the lid tightly. Steep 2-4 weeks, strain, and bottle. Label (example, fresh: "Elecampane, 1:2 95%, 9.2021, My garden"; example, dried: "Elecampane, 1:5 60%, 5.2021, bought from the herb store").

Dosage is 15-30 drops, 3 times a day.

Elecampane tincture with decoction

Tincture the fresh root (see preceding recipe). After draining off the tincture, barely cover the spent roots with water in a pan, bring to a boil, and simmer 2-4 hours. Stir now and again, adding more water as needed. Strain through a coffee filter.

Simmer the strained liquid on low heat for a few hours to thicken. Add the thickened decoction to the tincture and label. Shake the bottle every month or two, and shake it again before use.

Use as you would the tincture.

Herbal root candy

    1 cup (250 ml) root powder, such as
      elecampane, licorice, echinacea,
      marshmallow, lovage, angelica
    1 tablespoon lemon juice
    herbal syrup

Powder and combine the dry roots. Add lemon juice, which adds vitamin C and helps disguise some bitterness.

Add enough herbal syrup to make a stiff dough. It should be thoroughly damp, but not so moist that you can squeeze liquid from it.

Make small balls from the dough or spread it in a ¼–inch (5 mm) layer.

Dry in an oven or a dehydrator, where the flies it attracts can't get at it.

Store in an airtight container and take as needed for coughs, colds, and sore throats.

WARNINGS

Don't use elecampane for a dry cough.

Avoid elecampane if you're pregnant or breastfeeding.

If you're allergic to ragweed or mugwort, use elecampane carefully. Don't use it if you have a sensitivity to it.

Too much elecampane can cause nausea, vomiting, and diarrhea.

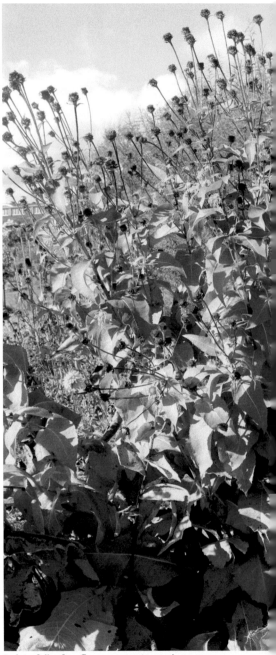

In late fall a few flowers remain on elecampane.

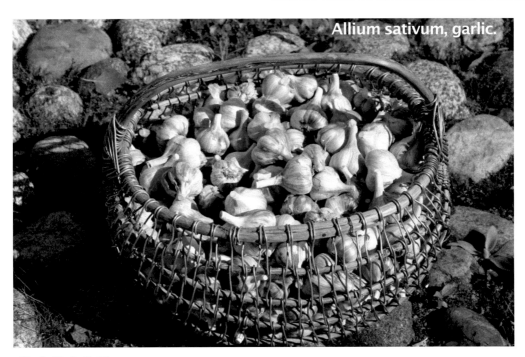

Allium sativum, garlic.

GARLIC

A really healthful stinker.

Allium sativum.

Other onions may be used, but they're a lot milder than garlic.

Taste: Pungent, aromatic.

Energetics: Warming, drying.

Family: Onion family, Alliaceae, or Amaryllis family, Amaryllidaceae.

Perennial: Cultivated as an annual or biennial. Harvest in fall.

Cultivation: Plant single cloves of hardneck garlic 4–6 inches (10–15 cm) deep in fertilized soil in September or October. Harvest full-sized garlic bulbs in late August the following year.

I prefer hardneck garlic, which keeps for about a year stored dry, to softneck garlic, which grows mold within weeks after harvest.

Grow your garlic in rows spaced 8 inches (20 cm) apart, with 4 inches (10 cm) between plants. If instead you tuck a clove here and another there throughout your garden, you may forget where they are, and you may not even notice your harvestable garlic growing between your lush late summer plants.

Harvest your garlic when the lowest leaf pair has turned yellow.

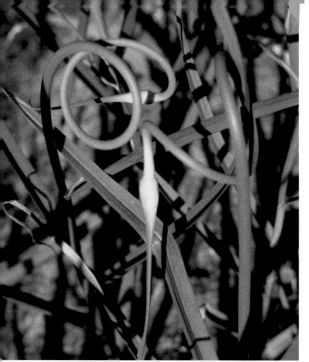
The fancy flower stalks of hardneck garlic.

Removing the flower stalks (scapes) doesn't really affect bulb size at harvest time.

The bulblets at the top of the flower stalks can be used like garlic. If you plant them in autumn, they'll grow into single cloves by the end of the following summer, and into full-sized bulbs one summer later.

For a winter garlic harvest, plant a few garlic cloves about 2 inches (5 cm) deep in a pot on a windowsill. Snip the greens as they appear to use in your cooking. (A windowsill clove won't grow into a bulb unless its pot is huge.)

Appearance: Garlic bulbs can grow to fist size, with numerous fingertip-sized cloves. The bulbs are covered in layers of papery, pale skin, the cloves in a tougher, usually red-brown membrane.

Important constituents: Garlic contains alliin (a sulphur compound) and alliinase (an enzyme needed to convert alliin into allicin); vitamins A, B1, and C; flavonoids; saponins; and trace elements.

PICKING AND PROCESSING

Dry freshly dug garlic bulbs as you would onions, in well-venitilated spot.

Dried hardneck garlic can be braided and used for many months. Softneck garlic grows mold fairly quickly at room temperature.

Use peeled garlic cloves to make tea, tincture, syrup, honey, vinegar, and infused oil.

Garlic will treat infectious diseases more effectively if you first crush the peeled cloves, and then leave them for a minute or two to give the alliin time to turn into allicin.

Simply munching whole garlic cloves will provide no allicin, which will soften garlic's impact on your flu or other infectious ailment.

Commercial "odorless" garlic products won't work very well for respiratory troubles, but they will strengthen the heart and blood vessels.

EFFECTS AND USES

Garlic is a warm, dry herb.

It's excellent for cold, moist problems, such as chronic ear, nose, and throat infections.

It's excellent for hot and moist problems, such as productive (slimy) coughs, and sinusitis. Discontinue the garlic once the problem is gone.

Garlic doesn't suit hot and dry problems, such as dry coughs or very sore throats.

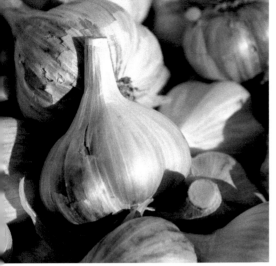
Garlic.

Garlic's heat and dryness is made milder when used in foods. Oven-baked garlic isn't all that hot and dry anymore. You can add fresh chopped garlic to yogurt, which is cool and moist. Garlic honeys and syrups are milder than garlic alone, and both vinegar and lemon juice make garlic less hot.

Garlic is first-class for treating lingering, productive (producing or coughing up a lot of mucus) respiratory tract infections.

Use garlic if you always get asthma when you get a cough.

Garlic strengthens the heart and blood vessels. Use it instead of a daily aspirin to help avoid another heart attack. Garlic has been shown to work better, and it doesn't have aspirin's side effects.

The elderly do well using garlic every day. It also strengthens the digestion and keeps infectious diseases at bay.

High cholesterol is a problem only if you suffer from familial hypercholesterolemia (FH)—hereditary high cholesterol. Cholesterol-lowering prescription drugs are life-savers for people who suffer from this problem.

Others will lower their cholesterol if they reduce their intake of simple carbohydrates (sugar, white flour, sweets, and so on), exercise, and take supplemental vitamins C and D. Add garlic to that, and your doctor shouldn't have to worry about your cholesterol levels.

Take garlic regularly to lower high blood pressure. You may even avoid starting blood pressure medication in the first place if you've taken garlic for months on end. Garlic may help you at least decrease your prescribed dosage, but first consult your doctor. It's dangerous to lower some blood pressure medications on your own.

Regular use of garlic (or onion) prevents some types of cancer.

You can make an infused garlic oil for earache, but where garlic takes a few days to stop the pain, mullein oil helps in minutes.

Garlic is useful for pelvic congestion. Try it for constipation, fibroids, cysts, and endometriosis, as well as for adhesions and similar scar tissue.

Dilute your garlic for external use. Crushed garlic can burn the skin. Hot herbs such as garlic should be removed at once if the skin reddens. Leave it on any longer and the skin will blister.

Instead, use a garlic compress, apply garlic oil (it smells terrible), or brush some garlic juice on the skin.

If you still wish to apply crushed garlic directly to your skin, first protect your skin with a cold-pressed cooking oil.

Raw garlic isn't for everyone, but prepared garlic works, too.

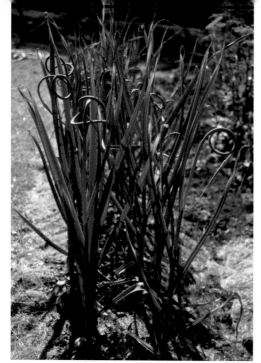
Two rows of garlic.

To prevent indigestion, give large amounts of garlic in increments rather than all at once.

Of course, those who are sensitive to garlic or onions should use other herbs. For most people, though, both garlic and onions are excellent foods and medicinal plants.

Garlic honey

cloves of 1–3 garlic bulbs
½pound (350 g) organic honey

Cover the peeled and crushed garlic cloves with honey in a jar. Add more honey the following day, if necessary. Cover and let steep 2–4 weeks.

Take 2–3 tablespoonfuls a day for asthma, allergies, coughs and the flu.

Simply garlic

Crush a garlic clove and leave it for about 5 minutes. Eat the clove, and then chase it with a drink of water.

Lemony garlic tea

1–3 crushed or sliced garlic cloves
1 tablespoon organic honey
1 teaspoon lemon juice
1 cup (250 ml) boiling water

Pour boiling water over the other ingredients in a mug, cool to a drinkable temperature, and drink. (Go ahead and eat the garlic pieces at the bottom, if you want.)

This lemon–honey–garlictea is very tasty.

Garlic syrup

garlic cloves
sugar

Crush peeled garlic cloves, cover with sugar, and leave overnight.

Take 2–3 tablespoonfuls a day for long-standing respiratory infections.

Don't use it for dry coughs!

Garlic vinegar

1 garlic clove
apple cider vinegar

Peel and crush the garlic clove, cover with vinegar, and steep for 5 minutes.

Eat the vinegared clove.

You can make garlic vinegar for longer-term storage, but for that I prefer a garlic-vinegar syrup.

Garlic vinegar syrup

2 ounces (50 g) crushed garlic cloves
½cup (100 ml) apple cider vinegar
5 ounces (150 g) sugar

Add the peeled crushed garlic cloves to the vinegar and steep for 4 days. Strain and add the sugar.

Take 1–3 teaspoons as needed for coughs and colds.

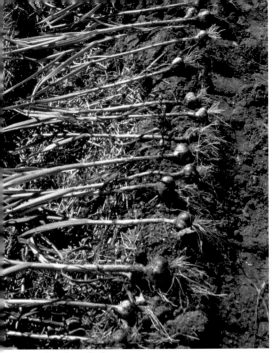

Hardneck garlic harvest.

Garlic oil

Make an oil from dried garlic (see recipe on page 7).

Massage the oil into the chest for colds and coughs, and massage into the belly for constipation, menstrual problems, and urinary troubles. (Caution: you will reek of garlic).

The oil is so smelly I can't recommend making it into a salve.

Fresh garlic oil

1 tablespoon garlic juice
1 tablespoon cooking oil

Mix. Put 2-3 drops in or behind the ear, if you don't have mullein oil.

Try garlic oil for hearing loss, as well. Dip a cotton swab in a little garlic oil and put it into the affected ear a few times a day. (Don't force a swab into the ear canal!)

Add more cooking oil if this mix burns!

Garlic tincture

From fresh garlic:
4 ounces (100 g) fresh garlic
8 fluid ounces (200 ml) 190 proof
grain alcohol (95%)

From dried garlic:
4 ounces (100 g) dried garlic
20 fluid ounces (500 ml) 120 proof
grain alcohol (60%)

Cover the peeled crushed garlic cloves with alcohol in a glass jar, and close the lid tightly. Steep 2-4 weeks, strain, bottle, and label (example, fresh: "Garlic, 1:2 95%, 7.2021, store-bought"; example, dried: "Garlic, 1:5 60%, 12.2021, farmer's market").

Dosage is 15-40 drops, 1-3 times a day.

Garlic compress

1 bulb garlic
1 quart (1 liter) water

Pour boiling water over the crushed peeled garlic cloves, steep 15 minutes, strain, and cool to just skin-comfortable. Dip a cloth in the tea, and squeeze out excess liquid. Keep the moist, hot towel on the chest (for coughs) or belly (for menstrual, digestive, or urinary problems) for 30-40 minutes.

Don't use garlic compress for inflammations.

This compress reeks of garlic.

THE SMELL OF GARLIC

If you eat garlic or use it externally, your skin, breath, and sweat will smell of garlic.

If you eat raw garlic cloves every day, however, after about three weeks the garlic smell stops.

Of course, another way to avoid trouble is to feed garlic to all your friends, as well.

Tricks such as eating an apple or parsley along with garlic don't work.

The smell is necessary to garlic's activity against infectious diseases. (One reason is surely that no one will come near you.)

Commercial, odorless garlic preparations are still effective in strengthening the heart and blood vessels.

FOOD USES

Make aioli—a garlic mayonnaise. Add garlic to stews, soups and casseroles.

Roasted garlic is a real treat.

Make a garlic soup, and try garlic ice cream (at least once!).

Make and use a strong garlic vinegar in your cooking.

Rub a split clove inside your salad bowl before adding the salad to add a hint of garlic.

OTHER USES

My grandma was told that garlic plants repel moles, so she planted it all over her garden. As it turned out, the moles loved the garlic. She said she thought they used it to season the flower bulbs they ate.

Try garlic water to repel insects that damage your vegetables: add 2 ounces (50 g) crushed garlic cloves to 5 quarts (liters) boiling water. Steep overnight, strain, and spray on your plants. (Don't do this for your leaf greens!)

WARNINGS

Don't use garlic if you take anticoagulants: the combination significantly increases a risk for bleeding.

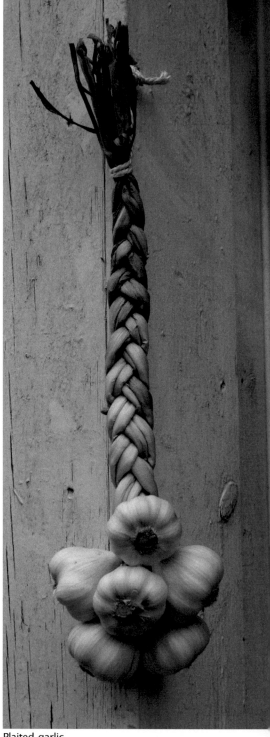
Plaited garlic.

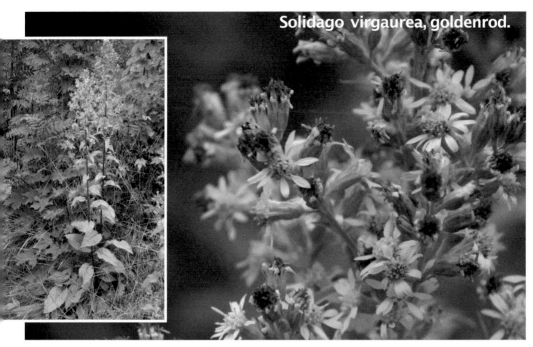

Solidago virgaurea, goldenrod.

GOLDENROD

Great both for urinary tract problems and for asthma and coughs.

Solidago virgaurea: Also called European goldenrod, Aaron's rod, woundwort.

Other species of Solidago with aromatic leaves among the flowers can be used, as well.

Taste: The topmost leaf is aromatic; leaves beneath the flowers are bitter.

Energetics: Warming, drying.

Family: Daisy family, Asteraceae.

Perennial: Harvest from summer to fall.

Habitat: European goldenrod is one of the first plants to flourish in logged-over areas. As the replanted area recovers, goldenrod hangs on along the edges of the woods and in sunnier forest meadows.

Imported species thrive along roadsides and meadows, as well as in gardens, where their flowers add a splash of yellow as the green of other plants fades.

Cultivation: Canada and giant goldenrods (Solidago canadensis, S. gigantea) are tall, fall-flowering perennials easily grown from seed. Readily invasive, these goldenrods will take over large areas of the garden and escape into other areas. Think carefully about where you decide to release them!

Appearance: European goldenrod has an almost candle-like inflorescence.

70

The flowers of giant and Canada goldenrod are quite showy, although their single flower strands go irregularly sideways. Most goldenrods have yellow flowers.

The underside of the European goldenrod leaf has a sparse network pattern.

Useful species have aromatic leaves among their flowers.

Important constituents: The flowering tops contain essential oils, tannins, saponins, glycosides, and flavonoids (such as rutin and quercetin).

PICKING AND PROCESSING

The stronger the taste of the topmost leaves, the stronger the herb.

Don't use mild-tasting plants or stands.

Goldenrod has a brief effective shelf-life. Pick new herb every year.

Cut or twist off the flowering tops beneath the lowest flower when the plants are in full flower.

If you want to keep the flowers yellow during drying, pick them while they're still in bud. Otherwise, your harvest will dry into brownish fluff. (Note, however, that the fluff works! It's just not as pretty.)

One European goldenrod plant can have up to several dozen flower stalks. Be gentle: if there are fewer than three stalks, pass the plant by. If there are five or so, take at most one. If there are ten or more, take at most a third of them.

Canada and giant goldenrod can be cut ruthlessly, as they spread ferociously. Cut every single flower stalk, or at least as much as you need.

A lot of plants resemble goldenrod—until they flower. You can harvest goldenrod leaf before the plant flowers if you know the plant well.

Drying: Remove damaged and dirty leaves and spread whole flowering tops to dry.

Flowers will turn to brownish fluff (seed) on drying. The fluff stays neatly on the stems and won't fly off into the world.

Pull everything off truly dry flower stalks and store your dried goldenrod in airtight jars. Label.

You can use asters (Symphyotrichum spp.) with aromatic leaves among their flowers instead of goldenrod. They, too, change to fluff on drying, and they, too, remain effective as fluff.

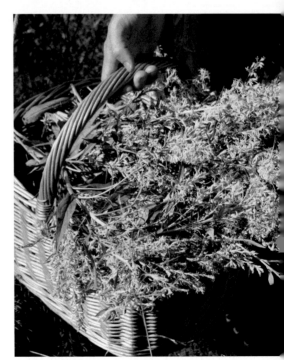

Goldenrod harvest in August.

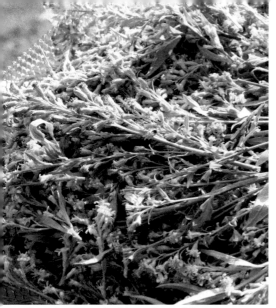
Flowering tops of goldenrod on a dehydrator tray.

Use goldenrod in teas, tinctures, oils, and salves. Decocting (boiling the herb) reduces its efficacy.

EFFECTS AND USES

The flowering tops of European goldenrod and other goldenrod species have been used for all kinds of urinary tract and kidney problems, from UTIs to kidney stones.

Goldenrod works nicely for urinary tract infections. To intensify the effect, add calendula and St. John's wort to your goldenrod tea.

Goldenrod can move stones from the kidneys to the ureters, where they can lodge. If you have kidney stones, see your doctor to learn the size of your stones before using goldenrod.

A goldenrod compress is useful for chronic kidney inflammation. Also drink the tea for several weeks. And visit your doctor.

Goldenrods are diuretic; that is, they increase the flow of urine. I don't use diuretic herbs as diuretics. It's better to determine the reason for the symptom, and then do something about that. Are your feet swollen because of a weak heart, weak digestion and liver, weak kidneys, or something else? Treat the cause of the symptom, and the symptom will go away.

Drinking the tea in the evening will have you peeing all night.

Use goldenrod for respiratory problems associated with asthma, hay fever, colds, sore throats, coughs, and even for the difficult breathing of emphysema.

A tea, tincture, or elixir of goldenrod is good for a dripping nose, especially if the drip is due to allergies. Add a few teaspoons of goldenrod tea to your Neti pot, as well.

Goldenrod can help with gout, rheumatism, and some other joint problems. If your joints are stiffer in the morning (even to the point of disability), the problem may be your diet. Go without solanaceous plants for a few weeks (which includes potatoes, tomatoes, bell peppers, chili/cayenne, and eggplant). Because potato starch, tomato, bell pepper, and cayenne are ingredients in a lot of foods, you'll have to make all your solanaceous-free meals from scratch.

Goldenrod leaves are styptic; that is, they stop bleeding. They're also astringent, so they'll remove excess water from boggy tissue. Try a tea of goldenrod leaves for heavy menses or for nose bleed, or give it for diarrhea.

Externally, a cooled leaf tea helps sunburned skin.

Gargle goldenrod leaf tea for sore throat, or use it to wash slow-healing wounds.

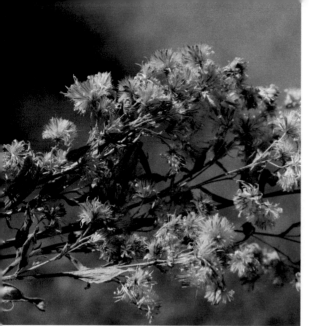
Goldenrod flowers change to fluff on drying.

The flowering tops are great, externally, for sore muscles. Try an infused oil or salve, rub in a liniment (a mix of oil and alcohol), or try a poultice or compress for locked-up muscles or a stiff neck. Also give it a try for muscle aches that nothing else has touched. (It won't help, though, with the aches and pains that accompany worn-out joints.)

A compress or fresh crushed leaves help heal difficult wounds and aching joints.

Use the infused oil for earache and tinnitus: massage a few drops behind the affected ear; if the eardrum is intact, put a few drops of the oil straight into the ear and seal it with a bit of cotton for an hour or so.

Goldenrod tea

1-2 teaspoons dried goldenrod
1 cup (250 ml) boiling water

Pour boiling water over the herb and steep 10 minutes.

Strain and drink 1-3 cups a day.

Goldenrod maceration

6 teaspoons dried goldenrod
2 cups (500 ml) water

Add herb and water to a pan, steep overnight, and sip this, cold, during the day.

Goldenrod tincture

From fresh herb:
4 ounces (100 g) fresh flowering tops, cut in ½–1-inch (1–3 cm) pieces
8 fluid ounces (200 ml) 190 proof grain alcohol (95%)

From dried herb:
4 ounces (100 g) dried flowering tops, cut in ½–1-inch (1–3 cm) pieces
20 fluid ounces (500 ml) 120 proof grain alcohol (60%)

Put the herb in a glass jar, cover with the alcohol, and close the lid tightly. Steep 2-4 weeks, strain, and bottle.

Label (example, fresh: "Goldenrod, 1:2 95%, 7.2021, Hillside Meadow"; example, dried: "Goldenrod, 1:5 60%, 12.2021, Mom's garden").

Dosage is 10–60 drops, 1–3 times a day.

Goldenrod elixir

fresh goldenrod flowering tops
fruit brandy or vodka
liquid organic honey

Fill a glass jar with crushed flowering tops of goldenrod. Add liquid honey to one-third of the jar. Then fill the jar with the brandy (or, in a pinch, vodka). Steep 2-4 weeks out of the light.

Strain, bottle, and label (example: "Goldenrod elixir, from plum brandy, 9.2021").

Take a teaspoon as needed.

Goldenrod oil and salve

Make an oil from fresh or dried flowering tops and make a salve from that (see the recipe on page 7).

Apply to painful muscles or joints.

Goldenrod compress

1 handful dried flowering tops
  or 2 handfuls fresh
1 quart (1 l) water

Pour boiling water over the herb, steep 15 minutes, strain, and let cool until just skin-comfortable. Dip a cloth in the tea, and squeeze out the excess liquid. Put the moist, hot towel on the hurt spot and leave it 30–40 minutes.

FOOD USES

Use the leaf in your herbal tea blends or include it in your green powder. Or add young leaf to salads.

WARNINGS

Goldenrod is diuretic; that is, it makes you pee. Don't drink goldenrod tea in the evening unless you like getting up at night to go to the toilet.

If you're sensitive to ragweed, mugwort, or latex, you may also react to goldenrod.

Large amounts of goldenrod can be toxic to sheep.

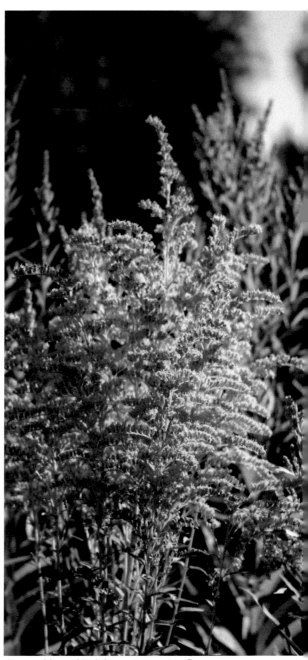

Giant goldenrod (Solidago gigantea) in flower.
Canada goldenrod looks a lot like it.

POTATO AND ITS USES

Potatoes are useful for a lot of things.

The liquid from a juiced or grated raw potato can help with heartburn and stomach ulcers.

To treat conjunctivitis, close your eye and apply some freshly grated potato. Leave it on for about 30 minutes. Repeat up to four times a day or until the inflammation subsides.

Remember: cleanliness is critical in all remedies involving the eyes. Don't touch the part of the potato mass that will touch the eye.

A fresh potato slice can draw splinters, thorns, and even a bee's stinger from the skin.

Try the boiling water of potatoes for frostbite. Boil peeled potatoes and use the cooled water to bath frostbitten toes or fingers.

Fresh potatoes have even been used as a local remedy for hemorrhoids. Fortunately, you won't have to use a whole potato. Instead, slice a suitable piece of a potato and apply it to the ouchy spot. Remove after half an hour, and repeat daily, until the need for a potato subsides.

Potato juice

1 peeled potato
water

Grate a potato, put it into a sieve and squeeze out as much liquid as you can.

Add two parts of warm water to each part of potato juice. Drink before meals.

You can dilute the potato juice with apple juice or similar, to make it more palatable.

It's a good idea to do something about stress, if the stomach problem is due to that.

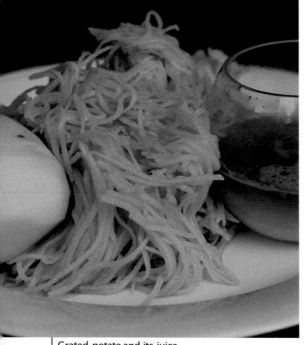

Grated potato and its juice.

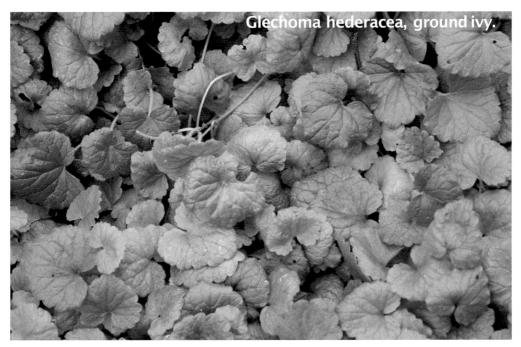

Glechoma hederacea, ground ivy.

GROUND IVY

Flowering blue in spring, ground ivy is a great herb for inflamed mucous membranes.

Glechoma hederacea: also called gill–over–the–ground, creeping Charlie.

Taste: Aromatic, mildly spicy.

Energetics: Warming, drying.

Family: Mint family, Lamiaceae.

Perennial: Harvest in summer.

Habitat: Ground ivy thrives in moist shady spots, where it will form a dense green mat in summer.

Cultivation: Move a few strands of ground ivy to a damp spot in your garden. Ground ivy is a low ground cover. It will grow roots wherever one of its leaf nodes touch the ground. You'll never get rid of it, if you plant it in your garden. Plant nurseries sometimes sell a variegated form of ground ivy. It can be used like the wild form.

Appearance: In spring, the leaves of ground ivy are only about ½inch (1 cm) wide. The small purple flowers appear in late spring in leaf nodes fairly close to the ground. In summer, the leaves are more than an inch (3-5 cm) across. Their taste is spicy.

Important constituents: Ground ivy contains essential oils, saponins, tannins (6–7.5%), bitter substances, and plant acids. The sesquiterpenes in ground ivy are not allergenic.

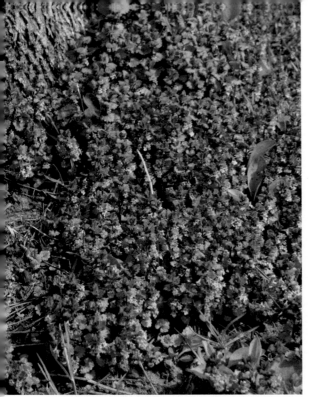
Ground ivy in full flower in late spring.

PICKING AND PROCESSING

Often, herb books advise to gather a plant in spring, when it's in full flower. It's far easier to pick ground ivy in high summer, however, when its runners have grown long and its leaves are fully grown.

To pick, grasp a handful of runners in the middle of a stand of ground ivy and pull gently. Break off runners here and there close to the ground and put your harvest in a basket. Repeat until your basket is full.

If your ground ivy stand is less abundant, take just a few runners from here and there, and then proceed to another stand.

Remove brown leaves and foreign matter, cut the runners into inch-long(2-3 cm) pieces, and spread them to dry. Store the dried herb in an airtight glass jar.

EFFECTS AND USES

Ground ivy is an anti-inflammatory plant in the mint family. It's excellent for inflamed facial mucous membranes.

Use it for inflamed or sore throats, for earache, tinnitus, and ear blockage caused by built-up ear wax.

Ground ivy is especially effective in noise-induced tinnitus.

It's good for both ear congestion caused by a prolonged cold or cough and for the prolonged cold or cough itself.

It helps with asthma. Ground ivy tea (strained!) in a Neti (nasal irrigation) pot can lessen or relieve headaches caused by sinusitis.

For ear congestion, try 3-5 drops of ground ivy tincture 3-5 times a day.

Ground ivy is a mildly bitter plant. Try eating a leaf or two 20 minutes or so before a meal to enhance your digestion.

Ground ivy's tannins make it useful for diarrhea (when taken internally) and for hemorrhoids (applied externally).

Mildly diuretic, ground ivy has been used for kidney problems and urinary tract infections.

Painters of yore often suffered from "painter's colic" caused by the lead in their paints. The tea, which is useful for lead poisoning, relieved this particular bellyache.

Some North American herbalists have used ground ivy to treat symptoms of poisoning from other heavy metals, including mercury.

Used externally, ground ivy treats bruises, cuts, scrapes, and other such minor skin problems.

Ground ivy tea

1-2 teaspoons dried ground ivy
1 cup (250 ml) boiling water

Pour boiling water over the herb, steep 10 minutes, strain.

Drink 1-3 cups a day.

For tinnitus, drink 3 cups a day until the noise stops.

Gargle the tea for sore throats, or add a little of the cooled tea, with salt, to your Neti pot.

Ground ivy tincture

From fresh herb:
4 ounces (100 g) fresh ground ivy, cut to ½-1 inch (1-3 cm) pieces
8 fluid ounces (200 ml) 190 proof grain alcohol (95%)

From dried herb:
4 ounces (100 g) recently dried ground ivy, crushed
20 fluid ounces (500 ml) 120 proof grain alcohol (60%)

Put the herb in a glass jar, cover with the alcohol, and close the lid tightly. Steep 2-4 weeks, strain, and bottle. Label (example, fresh: "Ground ivy, 1:2 95%, 7.2021, My garden"; example, dried: "Ground ivy, 1:5 60%, 12.2021, Bought").

Dosage is 1-15 drops, 1-3 times a day.

Ear steaming

1-2 teaspoons dried ground ivy
1 cup (250 ml) boiling water

Pour boiling water over the herb in a cup and steep 10 minutes. Hold your ear above the cup and let the steam caress it for 10 minutes.

Use ear steaming for tinnitus, earache, and congested ears.

Respiratory steam

1-2 teaspoons dried ground ivy
1 cup (250 ml) boiling water

Pour boiling water over the herb in a bowl, and steep 10 minutes. Breathe the steam 10-20 minutes to help relieve a cold, cough, or stuffy nose.

Ground ivy snuff

a pinch of dried, finely powdered ground ivy

Sniff the powder, and then sneeze. Use for sinusitis and congested ears.

FOOD USES

Ground ivy leaves add spice to salads, or add them to stews, omelets, soups or herbal sandwich spreads.

Cool ground ivy tea is refreshing on hot summer days. Sweeten it with honey, if you like.

WARNINGS

In large amounts, ground ivy is toxic to horses.

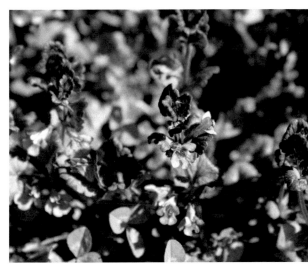

Ground ivy in flower.

HEARTBURN

Herbs give quick relief for some types of heartburn.

If your heartburn gets worse when you drink water, you have too little stomach acid. Stomach-acid deficiency is particularly common in the elderly. Take bitters 20 minutes or so before a meal to help remedy the problem. Bitters include dandelion, chicory, juniper berries (chewed), sage, burdock leaf, berberis, Angostura—and Campari.

If, on the other hand, a glass of water relieves your heartburn, you have too much stomach acid. Eat milder (less spicy) foods, drink less coffee, and above all reduce your stress.

You can, of course, also drink water.

The presence of Helicobacter pylori often is blamed for excessive stomach acid, but it's not the problem's root cause. Rather, the bacterium exploits a weakened digestion. You can get rid of it with antibiotics, but Helicobacter pylori will return fairly quickly unless you also strengthen your digestion.

Hiatal hernia can cause both heartburn and heart palpitations. Reducing stress levels helps reduce these symptoms.

Heartburn in otherwise healthy adults can indicate a food intolerance. You might find that your heartburn is cured simply by removing the offending food from your diet. First, do a test: eliminate the suspected food from your diet for two weeks. If your symptoms improve, you've pinpointed the cause of your problem.

Heartburn in pregnancy is caused by the growing baby shifting organs up toward the sternum. The pushed-on stomach has less capacity, and heartburn ensues. Eating smaller meals more often helps. Cooling foods and beverages can help, as well.

Reflux in babies is structural and very often normal.

Reflux in toddlers can be due to a food intolerance.

Heartburn can cause sore throats and hoarseness. Fix the heartburn, and the sore throat will be remedied, as well.

Heartburn can become chronic when the esophageal sphincter is damaged and scarred. It helps to eat smaller, blander meals more often.

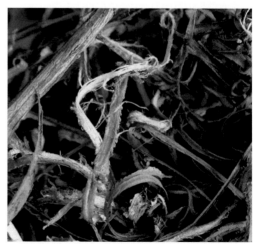

Barberry's yellow bark (Berberis spp.) is bitter.

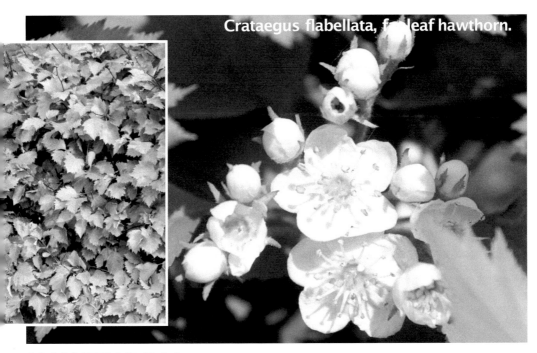

Crataegus flabellata, fanleaf hawthorn.

HAWTHORN

Stinky flowers, sharp spines, and mealy berries—but it's great for the heart.

Crataegus species.

Taste: The berry is mealy, a little sweet.

Energetics: Leaf and flower—cooling, drying; berry—moistening, cooling.

Family: Rose family, Rosaceae.

Bush or small tree: Harvest in late spring (flowering tops, leaf) and fall (berries).

Habitat: Hawthorn thrives in hedgerows, meadows, and forest edges. Various species are widely cultivated as hedges or small trees.

Cultivation: If you want flowers and berries, don't plant a hawthorn hedge. Hawthorns flower on the preceding year's branches, and in hedges, those will have been cut the previous summer. Trees, which are left to their own devices, produce plenty of both.

Appearance: Hawthorns flower in early summer. The flowers are about 1/3-inch (1 cm) across and grow in clusters. Flies and carrion beetles find the flower scent of some species irresistible. To us, they just smell bad.

The berries ripen in fall. They're usually red, sometimes orange or black. They're a little larger than the berries of rowan or mountain ash (Sorbus spp.) and contain 2-4 large, hard, angular seeds.

The leaf is round and often lobed or deeply cut. The leaf edge is serrated.

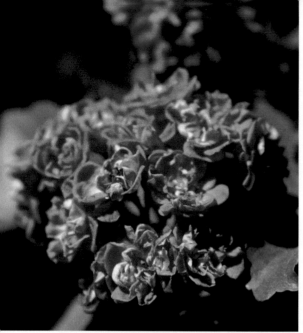

This pretty English hawthorn cultivar (Crataegus laevigata 'Paul's Scarlet') can also be used.

Along the branches are long (a little over an inch, or 3-4 cm), sharp, hard, often straight thorns.

Important constituents: Hawthorn contains many flavonoids (including 1-3% proanthocyanidins), which strengthen the heart and blood vessels. They're also antioxidant. Hawthorn also contains tannins, essential oil, vitamins B and C, fruit acids, and sugars.

PICKING AND PROCESSING

Europe's "official" species are English hawthorn or mayflower (Crataegus laevigata, C. oxyacantha) and common hawthorn or single-seeded hawthorn (C. monogyna), but all species work, including the black-berried Douglas hawthorn or black hawthorn (C. douglasii).

The flowers and white (or light pink) flower buds contain the most flavonoids, the leaf contains a little less, and the berries contain the least.

Although the flowers and flower buds are most efficient in strengthening the heart, it's a pain to gather them. Instead, pick the **flowering twigs** and cut them in 4-6-inch segments (10-15 cm) as soon as you spot the first flowers. If you're not fast enough, you may not get to pick any, especially if the summer days are warm. The flowers will be gone in just a few days.

In southern Finland, we have another problem in early summer, when aphids arrive on south winds. They love the tender young growth of hawthorn and will infest them all. They reproduce asexually, so don't pick infested twigs if you plan to dry your harvest. The amount of six-legged protein you'll find on your dried twigs will be unacceptable!

When picking the flowering twigs, wear long sleeves to slow down the thorns a little.

Tincture your fresh twigs, or dry them in a shady, well-ventilated spot on bedsheets, or use a dehydrator set no higher than 95 °F (35 °C).

Strip flowers, buds, and leaves from the dried twigs and store the material in an airtight glass jar in a dark cupboard. Label (example: "Hawthorn, June 2021").

Time saps this herb's strength, so pick new hawthorn every year.

Use dried hawthorn as a tea or tincture.

Pick **young leaf**, or check your neighbors' doings at their hawthorn hedges: help with the trimming, and then ask whether you may collect the leaves you need.

Harvest **berries** in fall, when they're fully ripe.

If the berries are soft when you pick them, process them into tinctures or elixirs as quickly as possible.

Hard berries can be split and spread to dry. Splitting them requires patience, a sharp knife, and sturdy hands. You might get blistered fingers, as the seeds are large enough to hamper your work.

Hawthorn's thorns are hard, straight, and sharp. Don't twist them from living branches to examine them. Remove them from a fallen branch, instead.

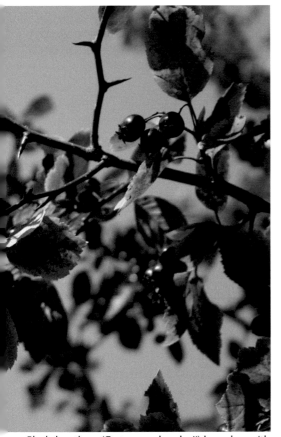

Black hawthorn (Crataegus douglasii) branches with berries.

EFFECTS AND USES

Hawthorn strengthens the entire circulatory system, from the capillaries to the heart. It soothes nerves, inspires courage, strengthens connective tissue, treats some inner ear problems, and can help some asthmatics.

If the berry is sour, it aids digestion.

Used regularly, hawthorn helps you better endure summer heat.

Hawthorn's astringent berries will dry boggy mucous membranes. To prevent it drying out the skin or eyes, add a moistening herb such as mallow leaf or psyllium seed, and/or mix the berries with honey.

The heart

Hawthorn flowers, flower buds, and leaves are great for all kinds of early heart problems.

Hawthorn

- strengthens blood vessels and capillaries
- strengthens the heart muscle
- improves the heart muscle's oxygen uptake and helps it use the oxygen more efficiently
- is a positive chronotrope (strengthens the pulse; that is, the heart pushes more blood per beat)
- slows the pulse (the heart beats slower)
- is a positive inotrope (strengthens heart muscle contractions)
- is a positive dromotrope (strengthens the heart's nerve impulses)
- is a negative bathmotrope (lowers the heart's excitability)
- enhances coronary and myocardial blood supply
- calms and relaxes

You can try hawthorn for congestive heart failure, but it won't help if the problem has persisted for a time and grown more serious.

Just a few decades ago, elders in northern England still chewed regularly on fresh leaf to strengthen the heart. There, the leaf was called "old man's sandwich."

Many herb books state that hawthorn starts to work only after a few weeks' of regular use. Happily, hawthorn hasn't read those books. It's immediately effective, at least for heart problems.

Hawthorn treats anyone with heart problems, except those who can't tolerate a slower pulse rate:

Some people may get palpitations, which are alarming. Others can't get up off their sofa. Both issues will surface by the second or third day of use, if they show up at all, and both subside within a day of stopping treatment.

A hawthorn allergy is very rare. Obviously, if you're one of the select few with this sensitivity, don't use this herb.

More serious heart problems

Hawthorn taken after heart attack accelerates healing and improves the heart's oxygen uptake.

Hawthorn is helpful in the early stages of congestive heart failure. Include it along with other medications—but check your medicine for side effects and incompatibilities.

Arrhythmia and irregular heartbeat

Hawthorn is excellent for irregular heartbeats, except in the few persons for whom it causes palpitations.

Blood pressure

Hawthorn affects blood pressure indirectly. Because it's so versatile in strengthening the circulatory system, it can help with high blood pressure.

To improve low blood pressure, I recommend a dietary change. Eat fewer simple carbohydrates and more greens, proteins, and salt. (A diet low in common salt is good for people who have high blood pressure, but not for those with who have low blood pressure.)

Exercise is great for both high and low blood pressure.

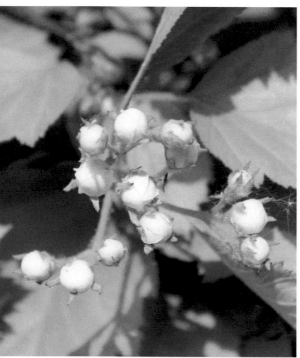

These flower buds of fanleaf hawthorn (Crataegus flabellata) will soon reveal their flowers.

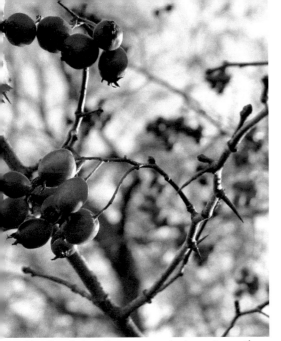

Hawthorn's long thorns are easier to spot once the leaves are gone.

Hawthorn and heart medication

Hawthorn is a good choice to treat heart problems in the early stages. The most commonly prescribed medication often addresses only the symptoms. Before long the cause will manifest in other ways.

Hawthorn strengthens the heart in many ways and makes blood vessels more resilient. This means problems resolve after only a few weeks or months of taking the herb. Hawthorn is harmless and nontoxic. You can start or stop taking it as you like, with no side effects.

You can take hawthorn for years on end, postponing the need for other medication.

Always consult a doctor if you have heart problems! If you think hawthorn can help you, discuss it with your doctor. If hawthorn improves your symptoms, ask your doctor to consider adjusting your heart medication.

Never stop taking prescribed heart medicine on your own. It can be lethal to suddenly stop taking a beta blocker, for example.

Cholesterol-lowering medicine, on the other hand, can be stopped without causing problems (unless you have familial hypercholesterolemia). Instead, lower your high cholesterol by changing your diet (fewer simple carbs are key here) and supplementing your diet with deficient nutrients (especially magnesium, zinc, and B vitamins).

In theory, hawthorn can amplify the side effects of beta blockers. In practice, this is rare, but know that the combination can lower your blood pressure a lot. Stop taking hawthorn if you start to feel faint, dizzy, or weak.

Nerves

Hawthorn calms, pampers the nervous system, improves mood, and slows down stressed and harried people a little and helps them breathe deeper.

Hawthorn is excellent for grief—good for the heart on many levels.

Hawthorn flowers and leaves act a bit more quickly than the berries, whose effects come on more slowly but last longer.

Use hawthorn in a tea or a decoction. Over time, if you take it regularly, it makes you less nervous.

Try a blend of hawthorn, rose, and milky oats for grief and anxiety.

Use hawthorn if you feel unloved.

Courage

Hawthorn gives courage. Try hawthorn, rose, or cinquefoil if you believe you're that timid mouse everyone uses as a doormat. You might be surprised—and surprise those around you.

The inner ear

For tinnitus, try ground–ivy(Glechoma hederacea) as a tea. It's especially good for tinnitus caused by long–term noise.

Or give a mix of hawthorn and ginkgo (Ginkgo biloba). Ginkgo strengthens the peripheral blood supply, and hawthorn strengthens the capillaries. The combination gets blood moving in stagnant spots such as the inner ear. Try making a honey paste from powdered ginkgo and hawthorn.

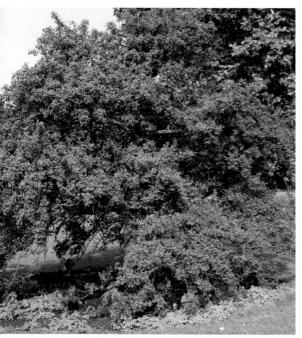

The branches of this tansy–leaved thorn(Crataegus tanacetifolia) bend under the weight of their berris.

The mix can also help with Ménière's disease, another problem of the inner ear. Add gotu kola (Centella asiatica) for more oomph.

Connective tissue

Hawthorn flowers and leaf, and to a lesser degree the berry, accelerate collagen generation, and thus strengthens connective tissue. This is why hawthorn is so useful in treating rheumatoid arthritis and tears in tendons and ligaments.

For these issues, it's a good idea to combine hawthorn with a mineral–rich herb such as stinging nettle or horsetail. For variety, use rose hips instead of hawthorn.

Digestion

If the hawthorn berry is sour, it strengthens digestion. A berry that's just "hawthorny"—that is, mealy and nondescript—will better serve the circulatory system and heart. A mealy berry is also astringent, though, and so can help with diarrhea.

Asthma

Although hawthorn may be useful in asthma, remember that asthma can signal the presence of mold in your living or working environment. Expect wonders only if the air you breathe is clean.

Asthmatics should also try a dairy–free diet for a couple of weeks. If symptoms decrease, continue for another six months. At that point, although hard cheeses or organic yogurt might no longer cause asthma symptoms, returning to a full dairy diet will only bring them on again.

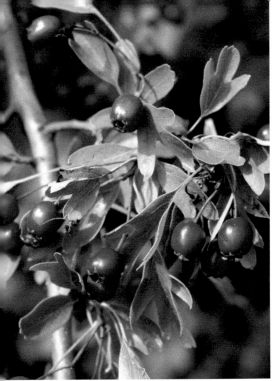

A branch of common hawthorn (Crataegus monogyna) in berry.

Hawthorn tea

1-2 teaspoons dried hawthorn flowering twigs, flowers, leaves, or crushed berries
1-2 teaspoons leaf or root of mallow (optional)
1 cup (250 ml) boiling water

Pour boiling water over the herb, steep 20-30 minutes, and strain.

Drink 3 cups a day.

Hawthorn berry decoction

1-2 teaspoons dried or fresh hawthorn berries
1-2 teaspoons mallow leaf or root (optional)
1 cup (250 ml) boiling water

Put plant material and water in a pan, bring to a boil, simmer 30 minutes, and strain.

Drink 3 cups a day.

Hawthorn berry tea

2-3 teaspoons dried powdered berries
1-2 teaspoons dried mallow leaf or root (optional)
1 cup (250 ml) boiling water

Pour boiling water over the herb and steep 15-20 minutes.

Drink 3 cups a day with or without straining out the herb.

Hawthorn tincture

From fresh herb:
4 ounces (100 g) fresh hawthorn flowering twigs, flowers, leaf, or crushed berry
8 fluid ounces (200 ml) 190 proof grain alcohol (95%)

From dried herb:
4 ounces (100 g) dried hawthorn flowering twigs, flowers, leaf, or crushed berry
20 fluid ounces (500 ml) 120 proof grain alcohol (60%)

Put the herb in a glass jar, cover with alcohol, and close the lid tightly. Steep 2-4 weeks, strain, and bottle. Label (example, fresh: "Hawthorn flowering twig, 1:2 95%, 6.2021, Karen's garden"; example, dried: "Hawthorn berries, 1:5 60%, 10.2021, Mom's house").

Dosage is 15-30 drops, 3 times a day.

To get all the various nuances of hawthorn in one bottle, make separate tinctures from flowering twigs, leaf, and berry, and then combine them.

To treat tinnitus, Ménière's disease, and similar inner ear problems. take 15-30 drops twice a day of tincture blended from equal parts hawthorn and ginkgo.

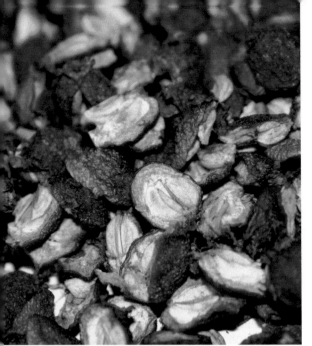
Dried hawthorn berries.

Hawthorn elixir

   fresh berries or leaves of hawthorn
   fruit brandy or vodka
   liquid organic honey

Fill a glass jar with the herb. Add liquid honey to one-third of the jar. Then fill the jar with the brandy (or, in a pinch, vodka). Steep 2-4 weeks out of the light. Strain.

Take one or two teaspoons as needed.

Hawthorn honey paste

   dried hawthorn berries
   dried horsetail or stinging nettle
   liquid organic honey

Powder the herbs (a coffee grinder is perfect for this). Add ¼-½cup (50-100 ml) honey to each ½cup (100 ml) powder. If you find this difficult to mix, warm the ingredients together in a bain-marie.

Take 3 spoonfuls a day to strengthen joints, tendons, ligaments, and other connective tissue.

Hawthorn ginkgo honey paste

   dried hawthorn flowering twigs, flowers,
      leaves or berries
   dried ginkgo leaf
   liquid organic honey

Powder the herbs. Add ¼-½cup (50-100 ml) honey to each ½cup (100 ml) powder. If you find this difficult to mix, warm the ingredients together in a bain-marie.

Take 2 teaspoons a day for tinnitus, dizziness, Ménière's disease, and similar inner ear problems.

A hawthorn bath

   water
   dried or fresh hawthorn flowering twigs

Fresh herb: Put herb in a pan and add water to cover.

Dried herb: Put herb in a pan and add three times as much water.

Bring to a boil, turn off heat, and steep 15 minutes. Strain. Add to bathwater with enough cold water to make a comfortable bath.

Get in and enjoy!

FOOD USES

Although our hawthorn berries are usually far too hard to be used like other berries, freezing them for three days or longer turns them soft and juicy. Now you can make them into jam, juice, and jelly. (Sometimes, but rarely, the berries are soft and juicy on the branch.)

Hawthorn is a great wine plant. Use either flowers or berries. The flower wine retains the taste of the fresh flower, while the berry wine is fruity and full-bodied.

Try small amounts of young hawthorn leaf in salads, or eat them straight off the bush or tree. Or add them to your herbal sandwich spreads. Consumed as food, hawthorn leaf will calm you and help you concentrate.

WARNINGS

Always consult a doctor if you have heart problems or vascular disease.

Never use hawthorn if it causes you to itch or stimulates other allergic reactions.

Stop using hawthorn if it causes palpitations or listlessness.

Hawthorn can amplify the side effects of heart medication. If this happens, stop using hawthorn at once. If you still wish to use it, ask your doctor to consider reducing the dose of your heart medicine.

Never reduce or stop taking prescribed heart medicine on your own!

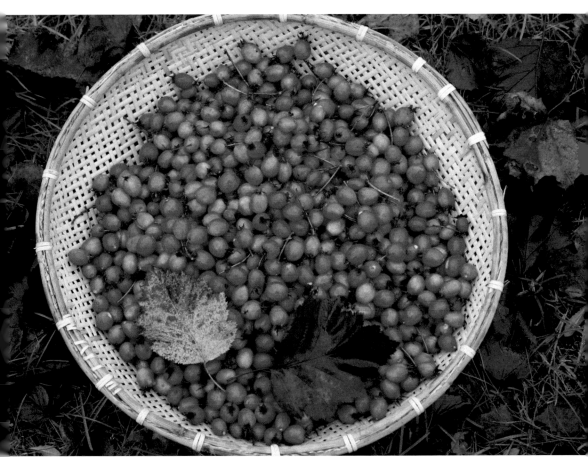

Ripe—but still very hard—hawthorn berries.

CABBAGE AND ITS USES

Cabbage leaf makes a nice poultice, and the juice is good for the gut.

Cabbage leaf offers quick relief for aches and pains.

For an achy knee, choose a suitably large red or white cabbage leaf and crush the largest leaf ribs to bring juice to the surface (a rolling pin is good for this), apply it to the achy spot, and leave it there 30–60 minutes. If the problem is minor, both pain and swelling will subside.

Cabbage leaves have been used by lactating moms for centuries to treat mastitis and other breast pains. Cabbage leaf comes in all cup sizes: crush a suitable leaf and leave it on the breast for half an hour. Of course, the best remedy for a mild breast problem is a nursing baby—the very best of breast pumps.

Don't leave the leaf on too long; it can suppress milk production. On the other hand, a cabbage leaf applied for an hour or two is great if you need to stop producing milk quickly.

Raw cabbage juice calms stomach ulcers.

Try the juice for irritable bowel or similar serious gut problems—but start with a small amount. If it helps, you'll soon feel excellent. If it causes twinges, gas, or diarrhea, however, cabbage juice is not for you. Give St. John's wort or mallow a try and leave cabbage juice to others.

Some people react badly to cabbage, but this is rare. Use other remedies if cabbage leaf makes your skin red and itchy.

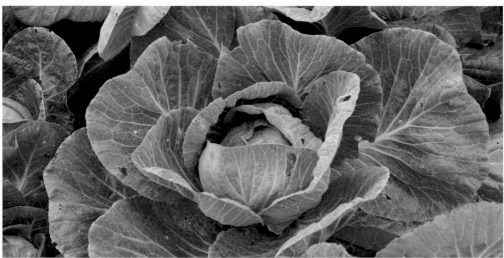

Cabbage leaves come in all sizes.

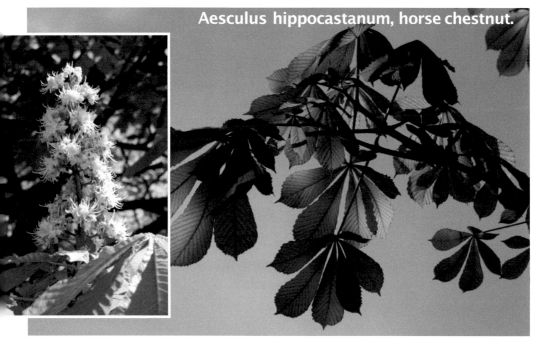

Aesculus hippocastanum, horse chestnut.

HORSE CHESTNUT

The inedible seed is a good medicinal herb.

Aesculus hippocastanum: Also called common horse chestnut, conker.

You can use other species of Aesculus externally, as well, but use them internally only if you know their dosage.

Taste: Biting, bitter.

Energetics: Warming, drying.

Family: Soapberry family, Sapindaceae.

Perennial: Harvest the leaf in summer and the seed in fall.

Cultivation: Plant seeds in fall to overwinter in pots dug into the ground. Then in the spring move the sprouted seeds with their pots to partial shade, transplanting to bigger pots as they grow.

After a few years, unpot and plant the seedlings in their final, preferably sunny, spot. Protect them from hares and rabbits.

Horse chestnut grows into a large, handsome tree.

Appearance: The flowers are gorgeous in early summer. The leaves are digitate (hand-shaped) and large. The fresh seeds are reddish-brown, surrounded by a spiky green shell.

Look-alikes: Chestnut (Castanea spp.) seeds are similar, but the seed shell is much spikier. Chestnut leaves are single, not digitate. Chestnut flowers are catkins, much like those of birch and oak.

Chestnuts are edible; horse chestnuts aren't.

Important constituents: Horse chestnut seeds contain the saponins aescin and aesculin, flavonoids, bitter substances, and tannins. The leaves contain aescin, aesculin, and tannins.

PICKING AND PROCESSING

Pick the leaves in summer and spread them to dry, or collect fallen seeds with their spiky shells in fall.

Cut the fresh seeds and their shells into ¼-inch (5 mm) slices and spread them to dry.

Seeds that have lost their glossy sheen will be too dry to slice.

EFFECTS AND USES

Horse chestnut strengthens the veins and treats stagnation. It's excellent for painful, achy hemorrhoids and varicosities, and for bags under the eyes.

Use horse chestnut for bruises, sprains, and scrapes to strengthen local blood circulation.

I mostly use horse chestnut for external treatment. Don't exceed the given dosages for internal use!

Oiled horse chestnut leaf

a single leaflet
fat or oil

Crush the leaf and spread some fat on its surface. Apply to the achy spot.

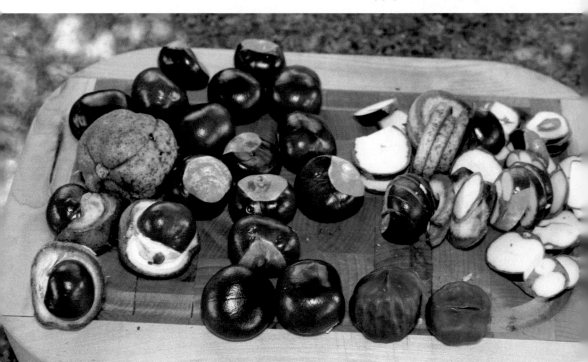

Horse chestnuts. The duller horse chestnuts in front are a week old and too hard to cut. The fresh ones can be sliced with a sharp knife.

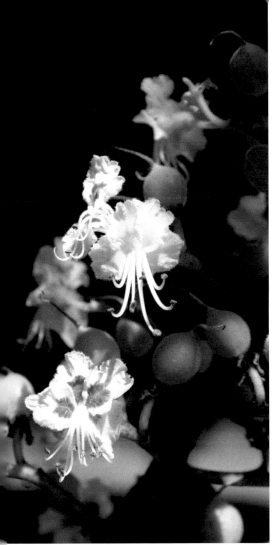

Horse chestnut flowers.

Horse chestnut oil and salve

Make an oil from dried seed or leaf, and then make a salve from that (see page 7).

I include dried young oak leaf and dried calendula flowers in my horse chestnut salves.

Apply the salve morning and night to varicosities, hemorrhoids, bruises, sprains, and scrapes. The salve also helps tighten bags under the eyes.

Horse chestnuts alone

People in some countries carry dried horse chestnuts in their pockets to ward off hemorrhoids.

Horse chestnut tincture

From fresh herb:
    4 ounces (100 g) sliced fresh seeds
    8 fluid ounces (200 ml) 190 proof
        grain alcohol (95%)

From dried herb:
    4 ounces (100 g) dried seed slices
    20 fluid ounces (500 ml) 100 proof
        grain alcohol (50%)

Put the seeds in a glass jar, cover with the alcohol, and close the lid tightly. Steep 2–4 weeks, strain, and bottle. Label (example, fresh: "Horse chestnut seed, 1:2 95%, 9.2021,Karen's yard"; example, dried: "Horse chestnut seed, 1:5 50%, 5.2021,Susan's garden").

Dosage is 1–5 drops, 1–3 times a day. Don't take more than that!

WARNINGS

They may look a lot like chestnuts, but horse chestnuts are toxic: never eat them!

Too much horse chestnut causes nausea, vomiting, and diarrhea.

Don't use horse chestnut internally if you take blood thinners or if you regularly take aspirin.

ONION AND ITS USES

A versatile medicinal plant.

The common onion (Allium cepa) treats a wide range of conditions, including cough (see page 125), earache, and urinary tract problems. In a pinch, it even makes a temporary bandage!

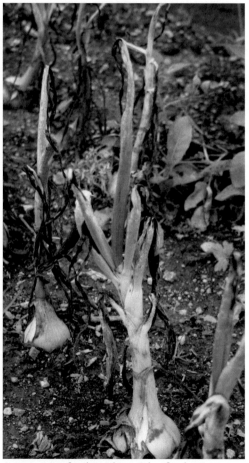

An onion ripe for the picking. Other food onions work, as well.

ONION FOR EARACHE

Use onions for earache when you don't have mullein oil on hand.

Fry a thick onion slice until it's soft, cool to a comfortable temperature, wrap in cloth, and lay it against the achy ear. Repeat as needed.

Or use the following home remedy—but only if the eardrum is intact: grate an onion and squeeze its juice through a cloth into the achy ear.

ONION BANDAGE

The membrane between onion layers makes a good impromptu bandage.

ONION FOR URINARY PROBLEMS

Eat a lot of fried onion if your urine isn't flowing as it should.

Or make an onion tea:

Onion tea

2-3 chopped onions
water

In a saucepan, add water to just cover the chopped onions. Boil 25 minutes, and strain.

Drink it all to treat the urinary retention of benign prostatic hypertrophy or the water retention before menses.

Don't use onion as a medicinal herb if you are sensitive or allergic to it!

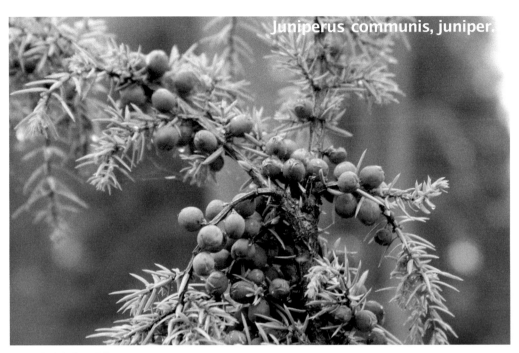
Juniperus communis, juniper.

JUNIPER

Juniper is a good medicinal herb—provided you don't take too much.

Juniperus communis: Also called common juniper, ground juniper.

You can use other species of Juniperus, but avoid savine (Juniperus sabina).

Taste: Aromatic, foresty. The berries are bitter, aromatic, and sometimes sweet.

Energetics: Warming, drying.

Family: Cypress family, Cupressaceae.

Bush or small tree: Harvest in fall (berries) or year-round (green parts).

Habitat: Juniper thrives in sunny dry spots in open pine forests and along the edges of dense deciduous forests.

Appearance: Juniper is a tall bush or small conifer. Its berry–like cones ("juniper berries") are black with a blue blush. It takes three years for the juniper flower to grow into a ripe cone or berry.

The needles are ½-inch (1 cm) long and very sharp. The wood is tough and scented.

Juniper grows very slowly. Some juniper trees are over 1000 years old.

Important constituents: Juniper berries contain essential oils, resins, bitter substances, and tannins.

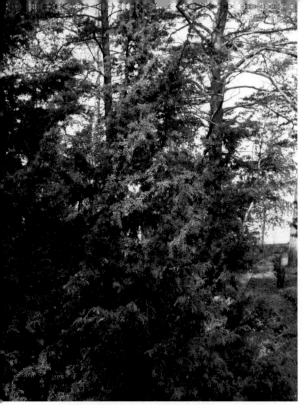

Juniper thrives in dry open forest.

PICKING AND PROCESSING

Harvest the berries in fall. Pass by junipers that still have green berries. It's a tedious process to separate unripe berries from ripe ones.

Use heavy gardening gloves and gather berries using a berry picker. It will fill quickly.

Or spread a bedsheet under the tree and shake the ripe berries from the branches.

To clean the berries, pour them at one end of a large terrycloth towel, and then gently lift it: the berries will roll to the other end, and debris will stay put.

Remove brown, green, and damaged berries.

Spread your blue or black juniper berries to dry, or dry them in a dehydrator below 85 °F (30 °C).

Because of their tough skin and high resin content, you must dry juniper berries three times longer than you would other herbs. Not-quite-dry juniper berries will grow mold very quickly in an airtight jar.

Juniper greens usually are used fresh, but you can dry them, as well.

Gathering prickly new juniper growth can be cumbersome and painful. Pine or spruce shoots are easier pickings!

EFFECTS AND USES

When you chew on juniper berries, you'll notice that bitters dominate. Used thus, the berries strengthen digestion and appetite.

Their essential oils are dominant in tea, and a hot juniper berry tea is good for coughs. The tea also is diuretic and helps with urinary tract infections.

Use the tea for gout: it helps remove uric acid from the body.

A juniper berry syrup treats coughs, colds, and flu, as well.

If you tincture the berries, resins will dominate. The tincture is diuretic and helps with urinary tract infections, but used long-term juniper berries weary the kidneys.

In his book Flora Fennica (1861), Finnish botanist Elias Lönnrot suggested a steam of juniper tea on the ears for hearing problems. He didn't specify how long to hold your ear above the funnel inverted over a cup of juniper berry tea, but I expect 10 minutes once or twice a day for a week will give some hints to its efficacy—or ineffectiveness.

Use juniper berries externally for aches and pains in your muscles and joints.

Juniper berry tea

1 teaspoon crushed juniper berries
1 cup (250 ml) boiling water

Pour boiling water over the berries and steep 10 minutes. Strain and drink 1–2 cups a day.

Juniper berry tincture

From fresh berries:
4 ounces (100 g) fresh berries
8 fluid ounces (200 ml) 190 proof grain alcohol (95%)

From dried berries:
4 ounces (100 g) dried berries
20 fluid ounces (500 ml) 120 proof grain alcohol (60%)

Crush the berries, put them in a glass jar, cover with alcohol, and screw the lid on tightly. Steep 2–4 weeks, strain, and bottle. Label (example, fresh: "Juniper berries, 1:2 95%, 9.2021, pine forest"; example, dried: "Juniper berries, 1:5 60%, 12.2021, bought from herb store").

Dosage is 20–40 drops, 1–3 times a day.

Don't use juniper tincture as a long–term treatment.

Externally, juniper tincture helps with muscle and joint pains. Massage it on the hurt spot, or make a compress:

Juniper berry tincture compress

2 fluid ounces (50 ml) juniper berry tincture
2 fluid ounces (50 ml) hot water

Combine. Dip a cloth in the tea and wring out excess liquid. Put the moist, hot towel on the hurt spot, eczema, or itchy skin and leave it there 30–40 minutes.

Juniper berry vodka

1 ounce (25 g) dried juniper berries
2 cups (500 ml) vodka

Put the berries in a glass jar, add the alcohol, and steep for a week, shaking it from time to time. Strain through a coffee filter.

Take a small glassful as an appetizer, or apply externally for sciatica or joint pain.

Juniper berry syrup

Make a syrup from crushed juniper berries (see recipe on page 1). Try adding some ginger to your boiling berries to spice up your syrup.

Take a spoonful of the syrup after meals.

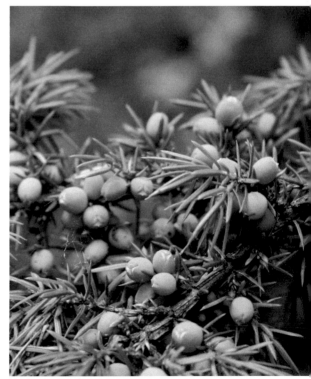

Unripe juniper berries.

96

A juniper berry bath or foot bath

1 quart (1 l) boiling water
4 ounces (100 g) crushed dried juniper
  berries

Put berries and water in a pan. Bring to a boil and simmer 15 minutes. Strain.

Bath: Pour into bathwater and add enough cold water to make for a comfortable bath. Get in and enjoy!

Foot bath: Pour into a basin and add cold water to a comfortable temperature. Soak your feet 10-20 minutes.

These help with joint and muscle pains.

FOOD USES

Don't use juniper in your food if you're pregnant or have kidney disease.

Use juniper berries as a spice for sauerkraut, pickles, sauces, marinades, venison, fish, fowl, beef, and the like.

Baked salmon is even tastier if you prepare it on a bed of juniper twigs (or other edible conifer twigs). Use your favorite recipe and bake your salmon skin-side-down on the twigs.

Tuck the twigs completely under the fish, especially if you use a hot oven (400 °F/200 °C). Otherwise, the uncovered twigs may catch fire when you open the oven door!

Use juniper bark or wood chips to smoke meat or fish.

Spatulas and butter knives made from juniper wood are beautiful and long-lasting.

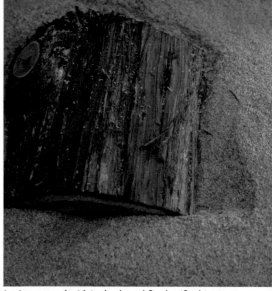

Juniper wood with its bark and finely sifted juniper sawdust.

OTHER USES

Juniper wood chips, bark, dried berries, and dried greens make good incense and smudges.

Well-sieved juniper sawdust makes an excellent deodorant bundle.

Juniper wood deodorant bundle

1 part sifted fine juniper sawdust
1 part sifted, finely ground blackcurrant leaf
  or 1 part sifted, finely ground elder flowers

Combine ingredients. Put a tablespoon of the blend on a piece of cheesecloth about 5 inches (15 cm) square. Gather the corners of the cloth and tie with twine to make a bundle.

Pat under the arms as a deodorant. The scent is gently masculine.

WARNINGS

Juniper resins can irritate the kidneys. Don't use juniper if you're pregnant or if you suffer from kidney disease. And don't use it continuously over a long period.

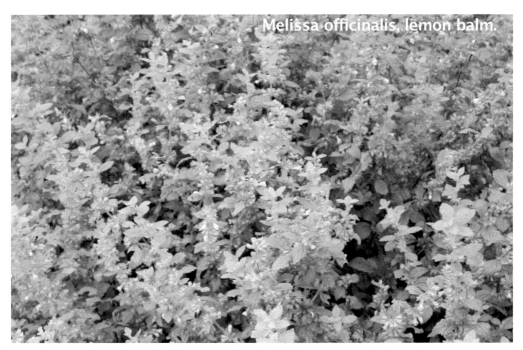

Melissa officinalis, lemon balm.

LEMON BALM

A very good herb for tension and stress.

Melissa officinalis

You can use lemon catnip (Nepeta cataria 'Citriodora') and Moldavian dragonhead (Dracocephalum moldavica) similarly.

Taste: Lemony, aromatic, a little bitter.

Energetics: Slightly cooling, drying.

Family: Mint family, Lamiaceae.

Perennial: Harvest from summer to fall.

Habitat: Lemon balm likes fertile soil in a warm and sunny spot.

Cultivation: Lemon balm is a short-lived perennial you can grow from seed or buy as a plant. It won't survive being covered by weeds.

If you buy lemon balm plants in the salad department at your grocery store and plant them in your garden, water the plants daily for the first week or two.

Appearance: Young lemon balm plants have rather large leaves, very unlike the small leaves of flowering lemon balm plants. The small white flowers grow in whorls near the leaf nodes.

Look-alikes: Young lemon balm looks a lot like stinging nettle (Urtica dioica), but stinging nettles sting. Look-alikes lack the lemony scent of lemon balm.

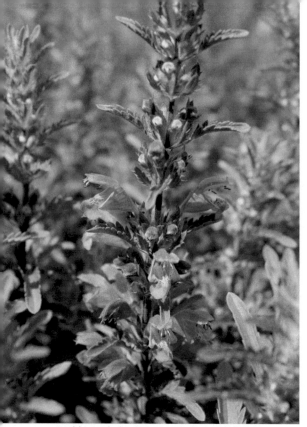
Moldavian balm (Dracocephalum moldavica).

Important constituents: Lemon balm contains, among others, essential oils (citral, geranial, neral, citronellal), tannins (as rosmarinic acid and other caffeic acid derivatives), and bitter substances.

PICKING AND PROCESSING

If the soil is fertile and the spot is sunny, you can cut 2 ft (60 cm) branches twice a summer. In poorer soil, lemon balm is smaller.

Gather flowering branches either before flowering or in full flower. The best harvest is in high summer on a sunny hot afternoon.

Strip the leaves and tops from the stems and spread them to dry. Or dry them in a dehydrator set no higher than 95 °F (35 °C).

Store your dried lemon balm in airtight glass jars. The dried herb will lose a lot of its scent in about half a year, but it will still work.

Use lemon balm fresh in teas or tinctures.

EFFECTS AND USES

Lemon balm reduces tension and nervousness. Use it for stage fright or prior to job interviews, for example, or give it to worked-up kids before long-anticipated events. (Take it yourself, if excited children stress you out.)

Lemon balm helps treat insomnia, palpitations, and stomach upsets caused by tension or nervousness.

It calms mild digestive problems. Try it for gas and bloating.

It's also of use in mild menstrual pain.

If you caught the common cold or have a fever, drink a hot lemon balm tea.

The French eau des Carmes (Carmelite water) was distilled from spirits, lemon balm, and spices. You can make your own similar, if milder, Carmelite brandy.

Externally, a crushed lemon balm leaf relieves the itch and pain of some insect bites.

A lemon balm bag under the pillow will help you fall asleep.

Apply a crushed fresh leaf or some (diluted) essential oil of lemon balm to quickly reduce cold sores.

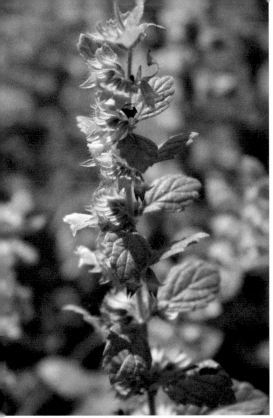
A flowering branch of lemon balm.

Lemon balm tea

1-2 teaspoons dried or fresh lemon balm
1-2 teaspoons mallow leaf (optional)
1 cup (250 ml) boiling water

Pour boiling water over the herb, steep 10 minutes, and strain.

Drink a cup as needed for nervousness, stress, and tension. Mallow mellows the tea a little.

Lemon balm wine

½cup (100 ml) powdered lemon balm
2 cups (500 ml) white wine

Put the herb in a glass jar, cover with the wine, and close the lid tightly. Leave for a week, and strain.

Take a small glassful in the evening for insomnia, or as needed for tension and nervousness.

Lemon balm tincture

From fresh herb:
4 ounces (100 g) fresh lemon balm
8 fluid ounces (200 ml) 190 proof
grain alcohol (95%)

From dried herb:
4 ounces (100 g) dried lemon balm
20 fluid ounces (500 ml) 120 proof
grain alcohol (60%)

Put the herb in a glass jar, cover with alcohol, and close the lid tightly. Steep 4-8 hours, strain, and bottle. Label (example, fresh: "Lemon balm, 1:2 95%, 7.2021, Susan's garden"; example, dried: "Lemon balm, 1:5 60%, 12.2021, bought from top herb grower").

Use 15-30 drops as needed.

Steeping the herb longer in the alcohol makes a good lemon balm tincture, but this quick tincture is exquisite.

Carmelite brandy

1 quart (1 l) fruit brandy (or vodka)
40 fresh lemon balm stems
or 100 g (4 ounces) dried lemon balm
1 lemon (organic)
1 tablespoon dried angelica root
2 tablespoons coriander seed
6 cloves
1 small cinnamon stick
1 teaspoon powdered nutmeg
or 1 nutmeg

Strip the leaves from the lemon balm stems, wash and slice the lemon, and slice or grate the nutmeg.

First make a lemon balm brandy: put lemon balm and brandy in an airtight glass jar, steep for 8 hours, and strain.

(If you're in a hurry, it's all right to strain the lemon balm brandy after 4 hours.)

Next, add the spices to the strained brandy, and steep 2–4 weeks. Strain through a coffee filter, bottle, and label (example: "Carmelite brandy, August 2021").

Take 15–30 drops in hot water as needed for respiratory tract infections or the beginnings of flu.

Or use it as you would lemon balm—for agitated sleeplessness, headache, palpitations, an upset gut, and minor menstrual cramps.

A lemon balm bath

2 quarts (2 l) boiling water
dried or fresh lemon balm

Fresh herb: Cover herb with water.

Dried herb: Put herb in a pan and add triple the amount of water.

Bring to a boil, turn off heat, and steep for 15 minutes. Strain. Add to bathwater with enough cold water to make a comfortable bath. Get in and enjoy!

A lemon balm bath calms and relaxes.

FOOD USES

Add fresh lemon balm to sweet foods, or (just before serving) to fish and fowl.

Use the leaves as garnish in cakes, beverages, and salads.

Or decorate water jars and pitchers with a few twigs of lemon balm.

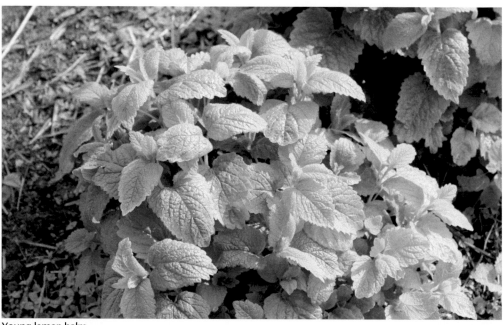

Young lemon balm.

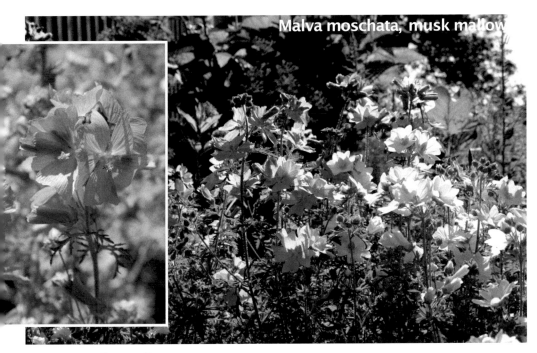

Malva moschata, musk mallow

MALLOWS

Good for mucous membranes and skin, but difficult to dry.

Malva species, including
- greater musk–mallow(Malva alcea), also called pink mallow, vervain mallow
- musk mallow (Malva moschata), also called white mallow
- common mallow (Malva sylvestris), also called blue mallow, cheeses or cheeseweed, high mallow, tall mallow

and close relatives, such as
- common hollyhock (Alcea rosea)
- marshmallow (Althaea officinalis); also called common marshmallow
- tree mallows (Lavatera spp.); also called rose mallows, royal mallows, annual mallows
- malope (Malope trifida)

I'll call all useful members of the mallow family "mallows."

Taste: Mild, sweet. Soft, unless the mallow is hairy.

Energetics: Cooling, moistening.

Family: Mallow family, Malvaceae.

Annual, biennial, and perennial: Harvest aboveground parts in summer and roots in fall or early spring.

Habitat: There are no wild mallows in Finland.

Cultivation: In Finland, annual mallow (Lavatera trimestris), malope, and common mallow are grown as annuals.

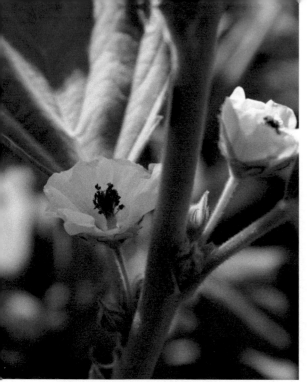

Marshmallow (Althaea officinalis).

In recent years, botanists have added several plant families to the mallow family. The old Mallow family, which includes the aforementioned species, is fairly straightforward. Its flowers all have a similar structure—five petals, five sepals, and one long pistil (the female flower part), with stamens (the male flower part) seeming to grow from this pistil. All mucilaginous parts of the old-fashioned mallows can be used.

Important constituents: Mallow leaves contain about 10% mucilage, some flavonoids, and a little essential oil.

Marshmallow roots contain 25-40% mucilage in fall. They also contain 5-10% sugars, about 10% pectin, an amino acid (asparagine), flavonoids, a hint of an essential oil, trace elements, and tannins.

Hollyhock is biennial; that is, it dies after it has set seed. Its close relative Antwerp hollyhock (Alcea ficifolia) is a perennial. Don't remove all flowered-out hollyhocks. Instead, wait until spring to see if there's new growth beneath last year's flower stalks.

Other perennials include the musk mallows, marshmallow, and garden tree mallow (Lavatera thuringiaca).

Sow seed outdoors in spring or early summer, or plant a seedling in a sunny, well-drained spot in lush soil. Marshmallow is true to its name: it loves wet feet.

Appearance: Hollyhock and marshmallow can grow to 7 feet (200 cm). Garden tree mallow and common mallow can grow to 5 feet (150 cm). The rest usually grow to 1½–3 feet (50–100 cm).

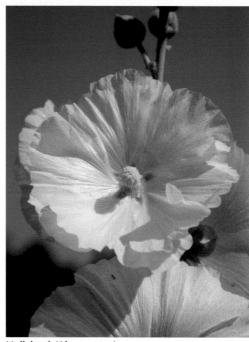

Hollyhock (Alcea rosea).

PICKING AND PROCESSING

Gather mallow leaf from early to late summer, when the plants are fully grown, healthy, and whole. Remove the stalks, which retard drying, and spread the plant material on a bedsheet, or use a dehydrator.

Cut the flowering tops of mallows when they start to flower to get another harvest in just a few weeks. Cut the tops into inch-long(2-3 cm) pieces, and dry them in a dehydrator set at 95 °F (35 °C).

I often find insect larvae in mallow flowers and unripe seeds. If you notice critters in your drying mallows, move your herb to the dehydrator. When they're well dried, put them in glass jars and then into your freezer for three days to kill any surviving larvae.

Remove the jars from the freezer, and put the plant material back into your dehydrator for a few hours to evaporate the condensed moisture.

Store your dried mallows in airtight glass jars immediately.

If you pick only the leaf, you'll avoid the bug problem, but you'll get less herb.

I find the only perennial mallow roots worth digging are marshmallow roots, which stay soft even when the plant is many years old. Other perennial mallow roots are woody and hard.

Prepare your dehydrator (or hot drying spot) before you dig your marshmallow roots. Efficient drying is essential. If the drying takes too long, these roots will ferment or mold.

Slice the roots into quarter-inch(5 mm) slices before drying. Remove the smaller roots and rootlets, which contain little mucilage.

Mallows are notoriously difficult to dry. They love water and rapidly absorb moisture from the air. If you can't use a dehydrator for all your mallow–drying needs, use one at least for finishing touches before you put them in airtight jars. Your mallows must be truly dry: they should crumble, not bend, when crushed, or your mallow will ferment or mold in its jar.

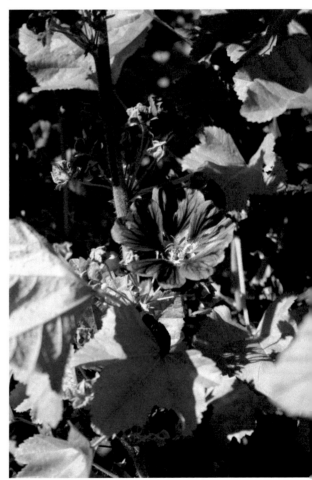

High mallow (Malva sylvestris 'Mauritiana').

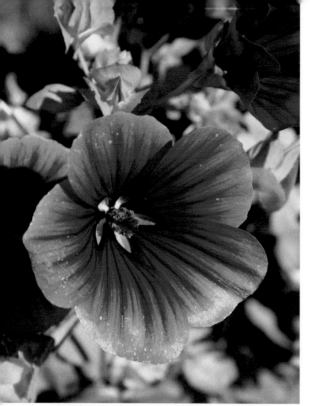

Flowering malope (Malope trifida), an annual mallow.

By far the most mucilaginous and water-loving mallow part, marshmallow root can contain 25 to 35 percent (and sometimes as much as 40 percent) mucilage.

Because the most important mallow constituent (mucilage) is water-soluble, mallows are best taken as teas.

If you must tincture a mallow, use low-proof alcohol. Strong alcohol renders the mucilage into far simpler carbohydrates.

EFFECTS AND USES

Mallows soothe mucous membranes. Drink mallow tea for long-standing digestive pain or diarrhea, a dry cough, a stuffy nose, kidney problems (and do visit your doctor for this), urinary tract infections, or just because your dryish mucous membranes need moistening.

Mallow mucilage helps loosen stuck mucus from respiratory tract and nasal membranes.

Try mallow tea for hoarseness. For throat problems, make a strong mallow tea, strain, pour it into a spritzer bottle, and aim the spray toward the back of your throat. You can, of course, gargle, but it's difficult to get the soothing tea where it's most needed that way.

After your throat spray or gargle, drink some tea, and then let your throat rest. Don't eat or drink anything for half an hour.

If your throat is sore because of heartburn, do something about the heartburn. In healthy adults, heartburn is nearly always a result of a food sensitivity. In Finland, the most common problem foods are gluten-containing grains or dairy.

Gargle a warm mallow tea to soothe inflamed gums and irritated membranes in the mouth.

Chew a chunk of dried marshmallow root to relieve sore throats, hoarseness, gum problems, and coughs.

A mallow syrup is great for dry coughs, but it lacks flavor.

Large marshmallow root pieces have been given to teething babies for centuries. The root is cooling and calming to inflamed, itchy gums.

Mallow teas help various urinary tract problems, as well as some prostate problems.

Mallow teas also can help relieve vaginal or anal itching.

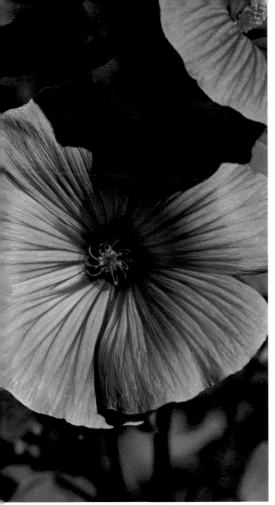

Annual mallow (Lavatera trimestris).

Add spearmint or peppermint to your digestive, respiratory, or urinary tract mallow tea for an even stronger soothing effect. Make a tea from the colorful flowers of hollyhock to vary the bland hues of mallow teas.

Mallows help "dry" people—those who drink a glass of water and then pee it out 10 minutes later. Drinking a tea of mallow leaf, flowering tops, or root for a few months can help them begin to retain water. Once they retain water, they'll have moisture to spare—they can sweat in summer heat, instead of fainting.

A dry person who also has low blood pressure (experiences dizziness when getting up quickly from a chair) should include more salt in his or her diet.

A mallow poultice or compress calms the skin. Use it for sunburn, mild burns, itchy eczema, or mosquito bites. Fresh crushed leaves or roots also work.

Use marshmallow root as a poultice or compress for bruises, minor burns, sprains, or strains, or on swollen wasp stings.

Take a mallow bath or sitz bath for hemorrhoids or vaginal troubles, to soothe your skin, or just to relax and calm you.

A marshmallow root decoction is useful for inflamed eyes. Strain it through a coffee filter, and make sure your procedure is sterile to avoid irritating the eyes further. Details follow.

A paste made from powdered dried marshmallow root draws splinters and such from the skin.

Mallow maceration

4-5 tablespoons dried or fresh
aboveground mallow parts
or 2-3 tablespoons dried or fresh
chopped-up marshmallow root
3 cups (750 ml) cold water

Add herb or root and water to a pan and steep 8-12 hours. Strain, or bring to a boil and strain.

Drink 2-3 cups a day.

For coughs, you may sweeten the tea, if you like.

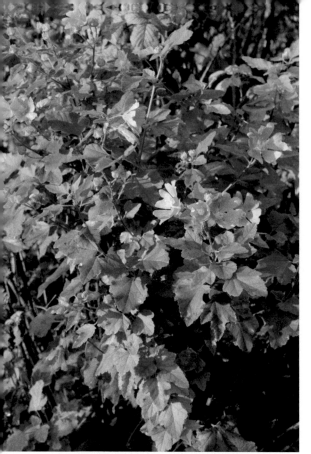

Garden tree mallow (Lavatera thuringiaca), a perennial.

A faster mallow maceration

2 tablespoons dried or fresh
aboveground mallow parts
1 cup (250 ml) cold water

Add herb and water to a pan, and steep for an hour. Bring to a boil and strain.

Drink 2–3 cups a day.

Mallow tea

1–2 teaspoons mallow dried leaf or
flowering tops
1 cup (250 ml) boiling water

Pour boiling water over the herb, steep 10 minutes, and strain.

Drink 2–3 cups a day, or moisten irritated skin with the cooled tea.

Marshmallow root decoction

2 teaspoons dried or fresh marshmallow root
1 cup (250 ml) cold water

Add root and water to a pan, bring to a boil, and continue to boil 12–15 minutes. Strain.

Drink 2–3 cups a day.

To make this into a compress for inflamed eyes, pour 1–2 teaspoons of the cooled decoction on a clean cloth and apply to the eye.

Don't touch the cloth on the side that will touch the eye.

Mallow syrup

Make a syrup from mallow leaves, flowers, flowering tops, or roots (see the recipe on page 1).

Take a spoonful as needed for coughs and sore throats.

Mallow compress and poultice

1 handful dried mallow
or 2 handfuls fresh mallow
1 quart (1 l) water

Pour boiling water over the herb, steep 15 minutes, strain, and cool to just skin-comfortable.

Compress: Dip a clean cloth in the tea. Squeeze out excess liquid. Fold and place the moist, hot cloth on skin that needs soothing. Leave it there 30–40 minutes.

Poultice: Fold 1–4 tablespoons of hot, moist herb into a square of cloth and put the poultice on skin that needs soothing. Leave it there 30–40 minutes.

A poultice stays hot for a bit longer than a compress.

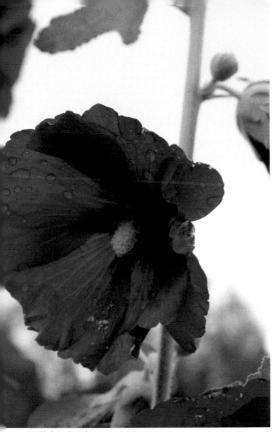

Hollyhock (Alcea rosea)

Mallow drawing paste

1 ounce (20 g) finely ground dried
  marshmallow root
2 ounces (40 g) cold-pressed coconut oil

Combine the ingredients in a small bowl until you have a fairly firm paste. If it's too runny, add more root powder. Too firm? Add more oil.

Scoop the paste into a small glass jar and label (example: "Marshmallow drawing paste, 3.2021").

Put ¼ teaspoon or so on the pad of an adhesive bandage, and put the bandage on the splinter for a few hours or overnight.

This works because the dry mucilaginous powder draws water—and with it any foreign objects—from the skin.

A mallow bath

water
dried or fresh mallow parts

Fresh herb: Put herb parts in a pan and add water to cover.

Dried herb: Put herb parts in a pan and add three times as much water.

Bing to a boil, turn off heat, and steep 15 minutes. Strain. Add to bathwater with enough cold water to make a comfortable bath.

Get in and relax.

Mallow tincture

4 ounces (100 g) cut-up fresh mallow parts
8-12 fluid ounces (200-300 ml) 60 proof
  grain alcohol (30%)

Put the fresh herb in a glass jar, cover with the alcohol, and close the lid tightly. Steep 2-4 weeks, strain, and bottle.

Label (example, fresh: "Marshmallow root, 1:3 30%, 9.2021, my garden").

Dosage is 30-75 drops, 1-3 times a day.

FOOD USES

Fresh mallow leaves added to salads and prepared foods, both salty and sweet, contribute "body." Mallows bring the same body to herbal tea blends.

Use smooth mallow leaves raw or cooked. Hairy leaves are better suited to cooked foods.

Decorate salads and cakes with mallow flowers.

Make a strongly purple tea from dark-colored hollyhock flowers. (Deep-red hollyhock flowers make a purple syrup).

Use it to color icings.

OTHER USES

Mallows make a moistening wash for dry skin.

Deeply colored mallow flowers change color depending on acidity or alkalinity. A strong tea will be brownish purple, but if you add lemon juice, for example, the tea turns dark pink. Baking soda, on the other hand, turns it greenish.

WARNINGS

All mallows are harmless.

Strain preparations made from hairy-leaved mallow species through coffee filters to remove hairs that can irritate tender membranes.

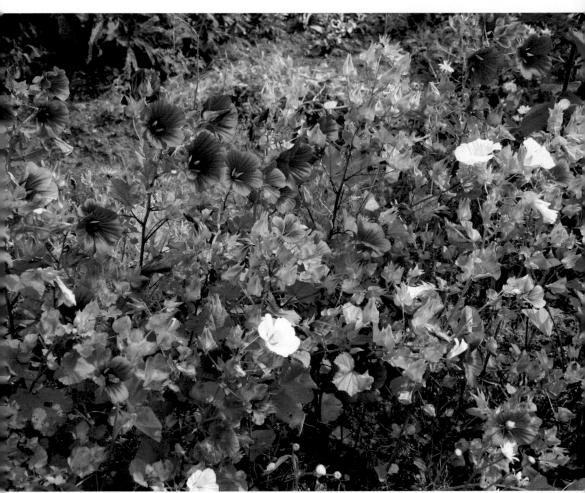

Pink-and white-flowering malope (Malope trifida)

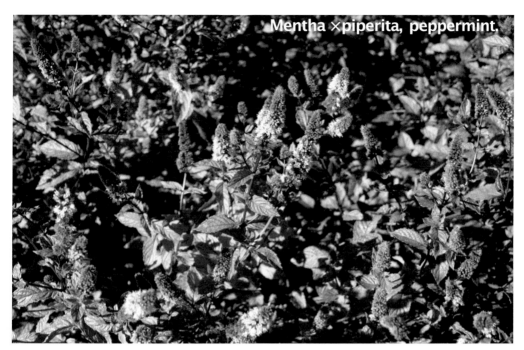

Mentha ×piperita, peppermint.

MINTS

Peppermint is both hot and icy cold. Other mints are milder.

Mentha species: These include pepperminty mints—

- peppermint (Mentha ×piperita, a hybrid of Mentha aquatica and Mentha spicata)
- Japanese mint (Mentha canadensis or Mentha arvensis var. piperascens), also called American corn mint, Canadian mint, Japanese peppermint, Chinese peppermint

and catnippy ones—

- wild mint, corn mint (Mentha arvensis)
- water mint (Mentha aquatica)
- silver mint (Mentha longifolia), also called horsemint
- spearmint (Mentha spicata), also called garden mint

- curly mint (Mentha spicata 'Crispa'), also called curled spearmint, crispleaf mint
- pineapple mint (Mentha suaveolens), also called round-leaved mint, apple mint
- pennyroyal (Mentha pulegium), also called European pennyroyal

Other plants often are called "mints," as well, such as catmint (Nepeta spp.), horsemint (Monarda species), mountain mint (Pycnanthemum spp.), and calamint (Calamintha spp.). Those with a pepperminty scent and taste can be used like peppermint; those with a catnippy scent and taste can be used like the catnippy mints.

I refer here only to true mints (Mentha spp.).

Taste: Pepperminty species are fresh and cool, catnippy ones aromatic (but not necessarily pleasant).

Energetics: Peppermint is drying and both hot and icy. Other mints are warming and drying.

Family: Mint family, Lamiaceae.

Perennial: Harvest from summer to fall.

Habitat: Our wild mints (wild mint, water mint) thrive in damp soil. Look for them in ditches, riverbanks, and damp meadows.

Cultivation: Only about 20 mint species come true to seed. The best way to get a mint you like is to plant a bit of root, preferably with at least one stem attached. Mint stems root easily, as well.

Because peppermint is a hybrid, all you can expect to grow from bought peppermint seeds is another hybrid mint or one of its parent species.

Soil affects mint flavor. A mint that tastes good might not when grown in a different spot.

Mints like dampness. One dry year, my mints emerged only after September brought a lot of rain.

Mint grown in a sunny spot will have a strong flavor and showy flowers.

Mints spread easily with underground runners that, in a vigorous stand, can grow to six feet (200 cm). These will produce new stands all over the place, so plant where you needn't worry about their invasive habits. Don't plant mints next to less exuberant plants. And don't plant the less aggressive peppermint next to another mint; it will lose out.

If you plant mints in half-barrels or tubs, fertilize them regularly. Mints "burn" the soil; that is, they take everything they need from a given spot, and after a year or two move elsewhere. Mint roots will escape through the drainage holes of shallow containers. (They'll escape over the edges, too.)

Mints hybridize easily. About 4,500 named mints exist, although if a Mentha connoisseur were to check them all carefully, it's estimated the number of "different" species would fall closer to 2,500. For instance, most Moroccan mints are curly mints. There are about a dozen curly mints, and some aren't spearmints, but peppermints.

Determining what any mint really is isn't a task for mere mortals.

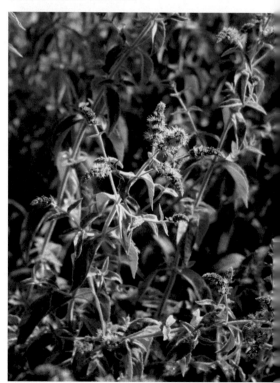

Silver mint (Mentha longifolia) in flower.

111

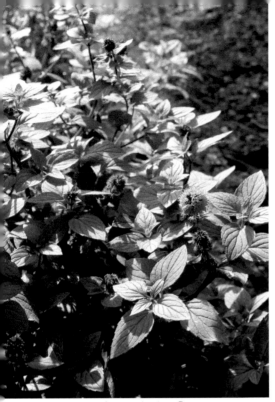

Water mint (Mentha aquatica) in flower.

To keep your mints true, remove any flowers before they produce seed. Otherwise, miscellaneous mints will sprout and mix with the original mint plants.

Appearance: Like other mint family plants, mints have opposite leaves and square stems.

Flower color ranges from light pink to dark purple. Some mints flower in spikes at the top of their stalks, others in small whorls around the leaf nodes.

Some mints are bald, others hairy.

Mints are perhaps most easily distinguished by scent.

Look-alikes: Many other mint family plants resemble true mints, especially before they flower. Check the roots. If you see a multitude of root runners, it's probably a mint.

Important constituents: Dried mint contains 0.5-4.0% essential oils. The essential oil of peppermint contains 30-50% menthol. The essential oil of Japanese mint contains 70-95% menthol. The essential oil of spearmint contains carvone (55-65%), and the oil of pennyroyal pulegone (85-92%).

Mints also contain tannins and bitter substances.

PICKING AND PROCESSING

Never pick endangered mints.

Many wild mints have the scent of cat pee. When I encounter these, I usually move on and look for mints that smell a little more pleasant.

When you find a wild mint that has a nice scent and taste, dig up a bit of it to transplant to your garden for easier harvesting in the future.

Take care to plant only mints that please you. Once they're established, they'll never go away. And remember—our tastes can change. A silver mint you loved five years ago may bore you now.

To harvest, cut the flowering tops two or three times a year, or pluck a stem as needed.

Dry in a shady, well-ventilated spot, either hanging in bundles or scattered on a bedsheet you've spread over a layer of newspapers.

Or use a dehydrator set no higher than 95 °F (35 °C).

Strip the flowers and leaves from dried stems and store the material in airtight glass jars.

You can tincture fresh or dry mints, or make syrups, oils, salves, or baths.

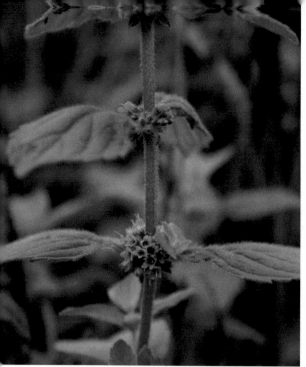

Wild mint (Mentha arvensis) in flower.

Use pepperminty mints as you would peppermint, and catnippy mints as you would catnip.

EFFECTS AND USES

Mints assist digestion, dispel gut and menstrual cramps, and help relieve coughs.

Use mints for bloating and gas, diarrhea, and respiratory tract problems. Try mint tea for nausea and vomiting.

Externally, a minty bath relaxes and calms. It also helps with menstrual or digestive pain.

A pepperminty bath peps you up and enhances peripheral blood supply. Try it for muscle and joint aches and for bruises.

Peppermints and spearmints cool and refresh. They're excellent for lung problems taken as teas, steams, syrups, or lozenges.

These mints reduce testosterone levels and enhance estrogen and progesterone in both men and women. Try them for hirsutism (lady beard): drink 3-4 cups of the tea a day. Men should avoid using these mints in large amounts, as they reduce libido and inhibit sperm production.

Take peppermint as tea or tincture regularly to help with smelly breath (halitosis). Its essential oil helps rid the esophagus of smelly bacteria. (If the halitosis is due to liver problems, help the liver instead.)

For headaches, fatigue, and migraine, moisten a cloth in peppermint tea or tincture and apply to the forehead. (For more about migraine, refer to page 26.)

Use the tincture in a homemade mouthwash (formula follows).

Oil or salve made from peppermint or its essential oil helps itchy skin, coughs (apply to chest and back), migraine, and joint or muscle aches. The salve cools and refreshes. It also repels mosquitoes.

Peppermint oil capsules are excellent for severe gut problems.

Externally, peppermint essential oil helps fend off oral herpes blisters if applied to the area before the blister has formed fully. (I'm not sure I'd apply peppermint oil to genital herpes.)

Mint tea

  2 teaspoons crushed fresh mint
    or 1 teaspoon dried mint
  1 cup (250 ml) boiling water

Pour boiling water over the herb, steep 5-10 minutes, and strain.

Drink unsweetened for nausea, gut pain, gas, bloating, or before meals.

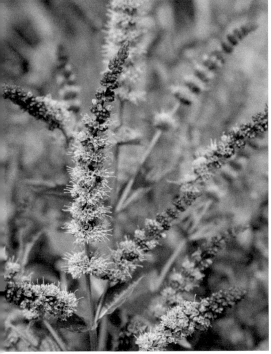
Spearmint (Mentha spicata) in flower.

Sweeten, if you wish, for coughs and colds.

For migraines, take a teaspoon of the hot tea every 10 minutes. (Read more about migraine on page 26).

Mint tincture

From fresh herb:
  4 ounces (100 g) fresh mint
  8 fluid ounces (200 ml) 190 proof
    grain alcohol (95%)

From dried herb:
  4 ounces (100 g) dried mint
  20 fluid ounces (500 ml) 120 proof
    grain alcohol (60%)

Put the herb in a glass jar, cover with alcohol, and close the lid tightly. Steep 2-4 weeks, strain, and bottle. Label (example, fresh: "Flowering peppermint, 1:2 95%, 8.2013, front yard"; example, dried: "Spearmint, 1:5 60%, 12.2021, Nan's garden").

Dosage is 15-30 drops, 1-3 times a day.

Peppermint mouthwash

2 tablespoons peppermint tincture
  (see foregoing formula)
4 fluid ounces (100 ml) 60 proof
  grain alcohol (30%)

Mix, bottle, and label. Add a tablespoon of the mouthwash to half a glass of water and gargle as needed.

A mint bath

water
dried or fresh mint

Fresh herb: Put herb in a pan and add water to cover.

Dried herb: Put herb in a pan and add three times as much water.

Bring to a boil, turn off heat, and steep for 15 minutes. Strain. Pour into bathwater and add enough cold water to make a comfortable bath.

Get in and enjoy!

Mint oil and salve

Make an oil from fresh or dry mint, and make a salve from that (see the recipe on page 7).

Peppermint requires around 10 percent more beeswax than other herbs to set properly.

Peppermint syrup

Make a syrup using the recipe on page 1.

A great variation on this formula uses 4 parts peppermint, 2 parts hyssop, and 1 part thyme.

Take a spoonful as needed for coughs.

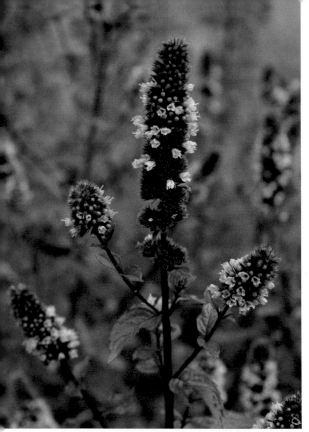

A strong peppermint (Mentha ×piperita 'Mitcham') in flower.

Peppermint capsules

vegetable capsules (available at herb suppliers, health food stores, and pharmacies)
1 tablespoon essential oil of peppermint
2–3 tablespoons oat flour
  or 2–3 tablespoons organically grown, non-GMO yellow corn flour

Combine ingredients in a small bowl, mixing well. Remove one end of a capsule, dip the longer part into the peppermint flour to fill it, and then close the capsule with the shorter end. Repeat until the bowl is empty.

Take 2–4 capsules for irritable bowel syndrome and similar severe gut upset, or take a single capsule as needed for less severe gut upset.

FOOD USES

Mint (especially peppermint) is a refreshing spice for greasy and sweet foods and for beverages.

Add mint to rhubarb pie, put a stem or two in your ice-water jar, put a few leaves in fruit salad, make mint sugar, use mint syrup on pancakes or ice cream, make your own minty ice cream, add mint to mutton or venison, make some tzatziki—or just enjoy a cup of mint tea.

Mint sugar

½ cup (100 ml) dried mint
2 cups (400 ml) sugar

Mix in a blender, strain, and pour into an airtight glass jar.

Use instead of normal sugar—for instance, in rhubarb pie.

Fresh mint sugar

½ cup (125 ml) tightly packed fresh mint
1 cup (250 ml) sugar

Blend until you no longer see single leaves. Use in desserts.

Store in the fridge, and use within three days.

Cool mint tea

1 teaspoon dried mint
  or ½ teaspoon crushed fresh mint
1 teaspoon dried organically grown orange peel
1 cup (250 ml) boiling water

Pour boiling water over the herb, steep 5–10 minutes, strain, and enjoy.

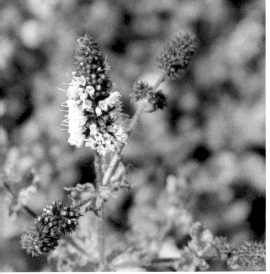

Curly mint (Mentha spicata 'Crispa') in flower.

Sekanjebin, an Iranian mint syrup

1 cup (250 ml) water
2 cups (500 ml) sugar
½cup (100 ml) apple cider vinegar
6 fresh mint twigs, 4-6 inches
(10-15 cm) long

Put water and sugar in a pan and simmer, stirring, to dissolve the sugar.

Add vinegar, bring to a boil, and simmer another 15-20 minutes. Add mint twigs and cool. Remove the herb, bottle, and label. Refrigerated, the syrup keeps for about a year.

To serve, pour 4-5 tablespoons mint syrup over ice cubes in a glass and top up with water.

Try adding a small grated cucumber to each two glasses of senkanjebin.

Tzatziki, or mint yogurt

2 cups (500 ml) full-fatyogurt
1-2 grated small cucumbers
or ½-1 grated long cucumber
2-4 tablespoons chopped fresh mint
garlic, salt, and pepper to taste

Mix. Serve cool on a hot summer day, or use it as a dip sauce.

OTHER USES

Peppermint-type mints are the most cultivated herb on earth. Their essential oil, or just their menthol, is used in toothpastes and mouthwashes, in candies such as chewing gum and chocolate, and to make menthol cigarettes.

Spearmint essential oil is used in sweets, as well.

Strongly scented mints repel insects. Use the salve against mosquitoes, or decorate your horse with mintsprigs to help keep flies and mosquitoes at bay. Decorate yourself, too, or the horseflies will try to bite you, instead.

Add a few drops of peppermint oil or peppermint tincture to a small spray bottle and squirt invading ants and their paths to put them off their scent.

Other insects depend on scent to find their prey, as well. Try mint on all of them.

Peppermint oil tick repellent

Make a spirit of peppermint:
1 part essential oil of peppermint
10 parts 190 proofgrain alcohol (95%)

Pour the essential oil into the alcohol, and mix.

Then, dilute it:
1 part spirit of peppermint
5-10 parts water

Mix, pour into a small nebulizer or spray bottle, and spray to repel ticks from dogs and people and horseflies and other biters from horses.

Do not use this on cats! They can't take essential oils, even in minute diluted doses.

Minty tooth powder

1 cup (250 ml) fresh mint, sage, and/or thyme
½ cup (125 ml) sea salt

Combine ingredients and blend to a smooth powder.

Store in an airtight glass jar. Sprinkle some on your moistened toothbrush and brush your teeth.

WARNINGS

In large enough amounts, ingested peppermint loosens sphincter muscles such as the esophagus (you get heartburn) and the urinary bladder sphincter (you dribble when you cough, sneeze, or jump—and, later on, when you walk).

If this happens, decrease your peppermint intake, do both pelvic exercises and squats to strengthen your pelvic area, and take mullein root tincture to help prevent urinary dribbles.

Don't use essential oil of peppermint undiluted, or you may develop a sensitivity to it.

Large amounts of any essential oils are dangerous to anybody.

Don't give menthol-y mints to babies. Their livers can process menthol after about one year of age.

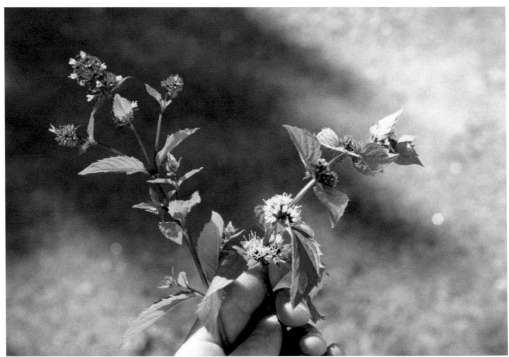

Peppermint on the left, Japanese mint (Mentha canadensis) on the right.

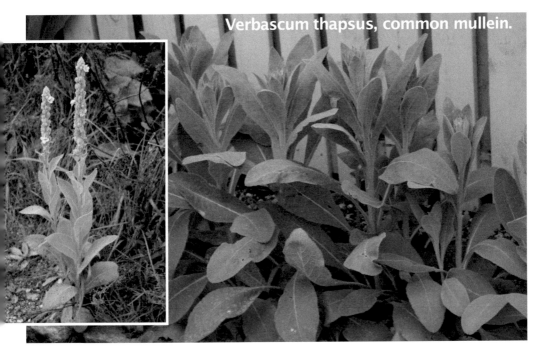

Verbascum thapsus, common mullein.

MULLEIN

Handsome plants with many uses.

Verbascum species: Among others, these include

- great mullein, common mullein (Verbascum thapsus), also called velvet plant
- dark mullein (Verbascum nigrum), also called black mullein
- orange mullein (Verbascum phlomoides)
- nettle-leaf mullein (Verbascum chaixii)

Taste: The leaf and root have virtually no flavor. The taste of dark mullein leaf is unpleasant. Mullein flowers have a sweet taste. All mullein aboveground parts are covered in itchy hairs, so use care when tasting these plants.

Energetics: Cooling, drying.

Family: Figwort family, Scrophulariaceae.

Usually biennial: Harvest in summer and fall.

Habitat and cultivation: Finland's two natives, common mullein and dark mullein, thrive in full sun in good, permeable soil, as well as on sand and in rock crevices. Mullein seed requires light to sprout. Covered seeds stay viable for hundreds of years. Dig where once there grew mullein, and you might find some growing there before too long.

Although mulleins hybridize readily, that doesn't matter for our purposes, because all mulleins are useful.

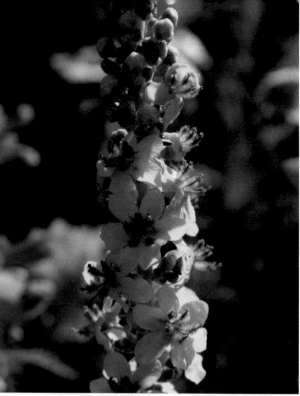

The flowering spike of dark mullein (Verbascum nigrum).

Most mulleins are biennial; that is, they flower in their second year. After the seeds have ripened, these plants die. The few perennial mullein species—such as dark mullein, purple mullein (Verbascum phoeniceum), and nettle-leaf mullein (Verbascum chaixii)—can be biennial, as well.

Appearance: During their first summer, mullein leaves sprout from the root to form low rosettes. If the winter wasn't too harsh, the plant will grow a more or less handsome flower stalk in its second summer.

Mulleins usually have yellow flowers, but white-and purple-flowered species and cultivars also exist.

Look-alikes: Less hairy mulleins can look a lot like toxic foxgloves (Digitalis spp.).

If you know both plants well, you're unlikely to make this mistake, but beginners should beware, and pick mullein leaf only after the flowers are visible.

Important constituents: Mullein flowers contain mucilage, glycosides, flavonoids, saponins and an essential oil. The leaf also contains some tannins, as well as potassium and calcium. The seeds contain a lot of saponins.

PICKING AND PROCESSING

Aboveground parts of mullein are covered in itchy and/or irritating hairs. Use gloves when handling large amounts of the plant, and strain all liquid medicines you make through a coffee filter.

Flowers

If you have a lot of flowering mulleins, you can pick single flowers without green parts. Use a wide basket; the flowers suffer if they're compressed.

Let the flowers melt into a clear liquid in a glass jar in a sunny window.

You can also use the flowers to make an infused oil or a tincture.

If you decide to dry your flowers, do it as quickly as possible. Set the temperature of your dehydrator (if you have one) as high as 140 °F (60 °C). Don't compress drying flowers, either.

Flowering tops

Cut the flower stalks below the lowest flower and either hang them up to dry, or spread shorter segments to dry in a dehydrator or on a sheet.

Once the flower stalks are dry, don thick gardening gloves (against splinters) and strip the flowers, seed pods, and flower buds from the stalks.

Use the stripped-off parts to make teas, infused oils, or tinctures.

Cut thinner-stemmed mullein stalks into inch-long (2-3 cm) pieces, dry, and use them as they are.

You'll also need garden gloves to strip the useful parts from fresh mullein stalks. Tincture the stripped-off parts, or dry them to use later.

Leaf

Harvest the leaf of dark-leafed mulleins only after they've begun to flower, especially if foxglove grows close by.

Gather light green (that is, hairier) mullein leaves when they're fully grown but not yet diseased or damaged.

It's best to pick mullein leaves off the flower stalks; they're high enough from the ground to stay mud-free in the rain.

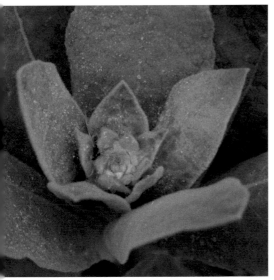

The leaf rosette of common mullein in spring, before flower.

If you picked mullein leaf in a rainy week, gently press it in a towel or sheet to remove excess moisture. Next, cut through the midribs of the larger leaves and spread them to dry, or cut the leaves into inch-long (2-3 cm) pieces and make a tincture or an infused oil.

Root

Most mulleins are biennial. You never dig roots of biennial plants when they flower, because by then the plant's energy has moved into the flowers. A biennial plant in seed is dying.

Dig the roots before flower, either after the plant's first summer or in its second spring.

Keep all good-looking leaves, and use them, as well.

Tincture or dry fresh mullein root. Cut larger roots into quarter-inch (5 mm) slices. Small roots can be dried as they are, or sliced once lengthwise.

Chew on the dried root or use it in teas and tinctures.

EFFECTS AND USES

Flowers and flowering tops

Mullein flower oil is an excellent remedy for earache. Use either the self-melted liquid you got from larger mullein flowers, or make an infused oil from the flowers or flowering tops. Drip one to three drops into the achy ear and wait for a minute or two, until the pain goes away.

Give mullein oil to children, as well. If the eardrum is pierced, rub a few drops behind the ear.

Otherwise, the flowers and flowering tops can be used like the leaves.

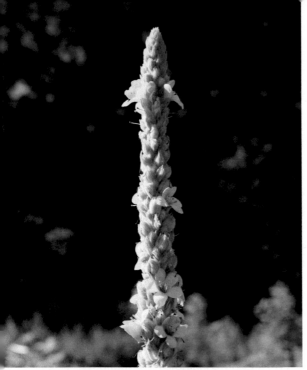
The flowers of common mullein.

Leaf

Mullein moistens and tightens swollen mucous membranes. Use the leaf in problems of the throat and respiratory tract. Give it in hoarseness and coughs.

Use the tea for diarrhea, and try it for colic and digestive pain.

Hold a candle under mullein leaf in a tea strainer and inhale the smoke just once or twice for asthma. This can stop an attack in its tracks. Keep your asthma inhaler (and/or goldenrod tincture) close by, though, just in case.

A little inhaled smoke can also relieve whooping cough.

For asthma, the long-term strategy is to take lung–strengthening herbs such as elecampane, mullein, sage (Salvia officinalis), and thyme. Add valerian or milky oats tincture to your blend if stress lies at the root of your asthma.

For asthma unrelated to stress, add hyssop (Hyssopus officinalis), instead. Garlic helps, if asthma always accompanies a cough or bronchitis. Almost all asthmatics fare better if they do without dairy: no milk, cheese, butter, yogurt, and so on.

Mullein tea helps when you feel as though someone is sitting on your chest and you have difficulty breathing. Take the tea in small sips until you feel better, and have your lungs (and possibly heart) checked.

Use mullein leaf as tea or tincture for hay fever, especially if you also have itchy mucous membranes and sneeze a lot.

For hemorrhoids, drink mullein tea and apply mullein oil locally, or use a mullein compress.

Add mullein leaf to your tobacco pouch to reduce your smoking. Add a little more mullein than before to each new pouch until no tobacco is left.

Apply mullein poultices for bruises, small wounds, and joint pain.

Root

Mullein root is good for incontinence. A few weeks of daily use leaves you much less likely to dribble when you jump, laugh, cough, or run. It's great for women who've given birth, as well as for the elderly, whose sphincters aren't what they used to be. The root strengthens the lower sphincter of the bladder, which we can't train on our own.

In addition to mullein root, do regular Kegels and squats.

The root helps other urinary problems, as well. Try it for urinary tract infections, inflamed testes, and bedwetting.

Herbalist Jim McDonald uses mullein root for spinal problems, especially if your back just won't straighten. He says to take a few drops of the tincture or half a cup of the tea, and stretch—and the back is straight. Herbalist Matthew Wood uses the leaf similarly.

The root can be used like the leaf and flowers for respiratory problems

Mullein tea

2 teaspoons dried flowers, flowering tops, or leaf
1 cup (250 ml) boiling water
1 teaspoon organic honey

Pour boiling water over the herb, steep 5-10 minutes, and strain through a coffee filter. Sweeten with honey.

Drink 1-4 cups a day for respiratory tract infections or the beginnings of cold and flu.

Drink 2-3 cups a day for a few weeks for asthma.

Mullein syrup

Make a syrup from mullein flowers using the recipe on page 1. Strain through a coffee filter.

Take a spoonful as needed for respiratory tract problems.

Mullein oil

Make an oil from dried flowers or flowering tops and make a salve from that (see recipe on page 7). Strain through a coffee filter.

Drip a few drops of hand-warmed oil into achy ears, or apply the oil to hemorrhoids or achy joints.

When using a pipette or eye dropper to deposit oil in the ear, never let any oil touch the rubber part. Oils dissolve rubber in just a year or two.

Clear mullein oil

Fill a glass jar with fresh flowers from a large-flowering mullein species and leave the jar in a sunny window for a few weeks. Add more flowers to the jar as and when you can pick them.

Little by little the flowers will "melt" into a clear liquid called "mullein oil." Strain this through a coffee filter and use as you would the aforementioned prepared mullein oil.

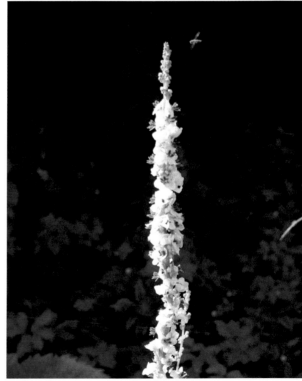

A white-flowering nettle-leaf mullein (Verbascum chaixii).

Mullein tincture

From fresh herb:
    4 ounces (100 g) fresh flowers, flowering tops, leaves (cut into inch-long(3 cm) pieces), or sliced fresh roots
    8 fluid ounces (200 ml) 190 proof grain alcohol (95%)

From dried herb:
    4 ounces (100 g) dried mullein flowers, flowering tops, leaf pieces, or root slices
    20 fluid ounces (500 ml) 100 proof grain alcohol (50%)

Put the herb in a glass jar, cover with alcohol, and close the lid tightly. Steep 2-4 weeks, strain through a coffee filter, and bottle. Label (example, fresh: "Mullein root, 1:2 95%, 7.2021, my back yard"; example, dried: "Mullein flowering tops, 1:5 50%, 12.2021, Zoe's garden").

Dosage is 5-30 drops (or less), 1-3 times a day.

Although mullein roots are white, the fresh root tincture turns a very dark brown within a few days.

Mullein compress and poultice

    1 handful dried mullein leaf
      or two handfuls fresh
    1 quart (1 l) water

Pour boiling water over the herb, steep 15 minutes, strain through a coffee filter, and cool to just skin-comfortable.

Compress: Dip a cloth in the tea, and squeeze out excess liquid. Put the moist, hot cloth on the affected area, and leave it there 30-40 minutes.

Poultice: Fold 1-4 tablespoons hot moist herb in a piece of cloth and hold it on the affected area 30-40 minutes.

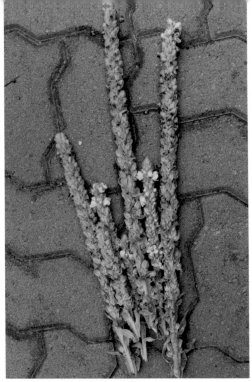

Common mullein flower stalks.

Mullein smoke

    small piece of dried flowering tops
    candle
    metal tea strainer

Dried mullein flowering tops won't ignite, so you'll need a candle. Put the mullein into a small metal tea strainer or sieve and hold it over the candle flame to make the mullein smoke.

A few short inhalations will halt asthma attacks and lessen ferocious coughing. The inhaled smoke should even work for whooping cough.

For children, the necessary dose of smoke is very small. Hold mullein over a burning candle in the room with the coughing child. Once you see just a wisp of smoke, remove the mullein from the flame. The smoke will promptly stop.

Dried mullein leaf burns well. If you use them, prepare to douse the flame.

Mullein milk poultice

1 handful dried mullein leaf
1 quart (1 l) milk

Simmer the leaf in the milk over low heat for 15 minutes.

Fold 1-4 tablespoons hot moist herb in a piece of cloth and hold it on the affected area 30-40 minutes.

OTHER USES

Dried mullein stalks dipped in flammable oils or waxes have been used as torches. I've tried to ignite dried mullein stalks without first dipping them in, say, tar, lard, or beeswax, but the stalks wouldn't burn. I'm told that larded mullein torches smoke and smell bad, and drip burning bits here and there.

Because mullein seeds contain a lot of saponins, historically they've been used for easy fishing. Fishing with saponin-rich plants is illegal almost everywhere it's traditionally been done. (Plus it's unsportsmanlike and unfair!)

If we grow gills, the seeds will stun us, too, but until we do, the worst they can do is give us a spot of diarrhea.

Dried mullein is said to repel rodents, but I haven't tried it.

WARNINGS

Strain all products made from the aboveground parts of mullein through coffee filters to eliminate itchy hairs.

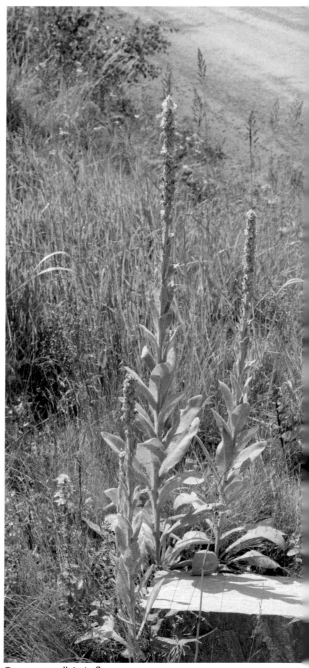

Common mullein in flower.

Vegetables:

ONIONS FOR COUGHS

Onions are great for coughs.

The humble onion helps even babies with stuffy noses.

A clean cotton sock stuffed with half a chopped onion and placed near the sleeping infant will keep baby's airways open when she has a cold or a cough. This helps baby and her parents to sleep better, the infection resolves faster, and the parents might avoid getting this particular respiratory tract infection.

Adults, too, sleep better when they can breathe through their noses and can benefit from an onion sock.

Onion sock

½ chopped onion
clean cotton sock

Chop the onion (no need to peel it), stuff it into the sock, and knot the open end. Keep the onion sock near the sniffly one's head as she sleeps.

Empty the sock in the morning, rinse it well, and hang it to dry. Use it to make another onion sock the following night, if necessary. Launder the sock when it gets too smelly.

Onion cough syrup

2–3 onions
white or brown sugar

Peel and chop the onions. Alternate half–inch layers of sugar and onion in a glass jar, starting and ending with sugar. Refrigerate overnight.

You can strain out the onions or leave them in the syrup.

Take a spoonful as needed for coughs.

The refrigerated syrup keeps for about a month.

A fast onion syrup

1 onion
sugar

Peel and slice the onion. Layer the slices in a bowl with sugar and leave for 30 minutes.

Take a spoonful of the resulting syrup as needed for coughs.

The onion slices can be used in pork or liver dishes.

Onion honey

1–3 onions
organic honey

Peel and chop the onions. Cover them with honey and leave overnight.

Take a spoonful as needed for coughs.

Avoid onions if you react badly to them!

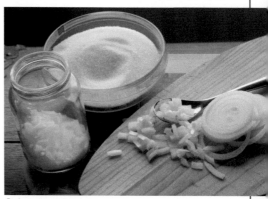

Onion syrup in progress.

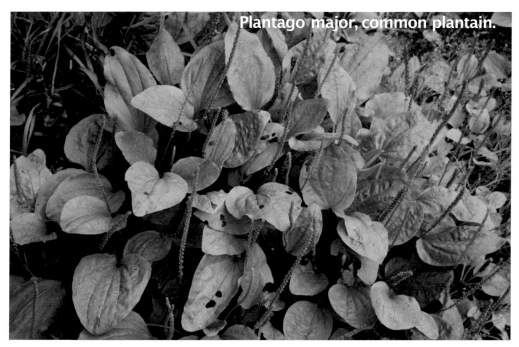

Plantago major, common plantain.

PLANTAINS

The leaf is good for coughs and small wounds, and the seed calms the digestion.

Plantago species: These include

- common plantain, greater plantain (Plantago major), also called broadleaf plantain
- ribwort plantain (Plantago lanceolata), also called narrowleaf plantain, lamb's tongue
- hoary plantain (Plantago media)
- sea plantain (Plantago maritima), also called seaside plantain, goose tongue

These plantains are not banana-type plantains.

Taste: Neutral, a little bitter.

Energetics: Cooling, moistening.

Family: Plantain family, Plantaginaceae.

Perennial: Harvest from summer to fall.

Habitat: Plantains grow almost everywhere, all over the world.

Common plantain thrives in yards and paths. It's small in dry spots and larger in moist, fertile soil.

Ribwort plantain will thrive in dry spots, provided the soil is not too acidic.

Sea plantain is common along the coast of the Baltic Sea. Look for it on other sea coasts, as well.

Cultivation: If you use a lot of plantain, consider growing ribwort plantain in rows. It's perennial and likes fertile, sandy soil in a sunny spot. Weed around your plantains, or they'll stay small.

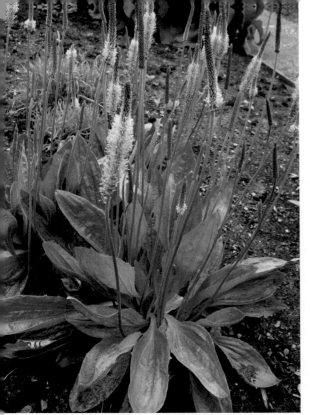

Hoary plantain (Plantago media).

Appearance: Finnish plantain species grow from a leaf rosette with flower stalks in the center.

The leaf veins of larger-leafed species are tough. You can see them clearly if you gently pull a leaf apart across the veins.

The flowers and flower heads of common plantain are an inconspicuous green. The flower heads of ribwort and hoary plantain are showy and white or pink.

Important constituents: Plantain leaf constituents include mucilage, tannins, flavonoids, allantoin (which speeds tissue healing), and the glycoside aucubin (which slows the growth of some bacteria).

Plantain seeds and seed coats contain mucilage, fat, and aucubin.

PICKING AND PROCESSING

Gather clean plantain leaves from summer to early fall, when they're full-sized but not yet diseased. Handle the leaves with care: bruised leaves turn black on drying. Blackened leaves still work, but they won't be as strong as they could have been.

Use your harvest fresh, or spread the leaves to dry in a shady, well-ventilated spot.

You'll often read that ribwort plantain is best. If it grew wild here, I'd say that, too, because you can gather a large basketful of ribwort plantain from a good spot very quickly. Just grab a large, tall ribwort plantain plant at its base, slice it off a little aboveground, and you're done.

Harvesting common plantain is a drag by comparison, especially in poor soil where the plants stay tiny.

EFFECTS AND USES

Plantain leaf soothes mucous membranes and calms inflamed tissues.

Use it as a tea, gargle, or syrup for dry coughs and hoarseness.

The leaf also helps with urinary tract infections and digestive problems such as diarrhea and stomachache.

Use it for insect bites and the itch from stinging nettles. Crush a leaf to bring its juices to the surface (or chew it—but don't swallow the juice!), and put the leaf against the itchy or irritated spot.

Small cuts and bruises heal faster with plantain's help. For larger wounds and cuts (incisions from an operation, for example), it's better to take plantain internally.

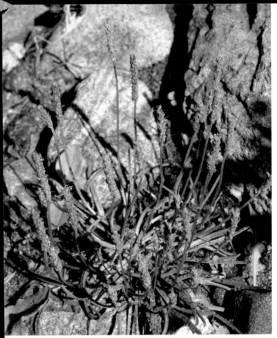

Sea plantain, Plantago maritima.

Crushed plantain leaf

Crush the leaf to bring its juice to the surface. Apply to the itchy or ouchy spot. Reapply as needed.

Plantain tea

> 1-2 teaspoons dried or fresh leaves
> 1 cup (250 ml) boiling water

Pour boiling water over the herb, steep 10 minutes, and strain.

Drink 1-3 cups a day for coughs, sore throat, urinary tract infections, digestive problems, or to speed recuperation from influenza or similarly sapping disease, operation, or injury.

Plantain leaf for acne

Crush the leaf (or use freshly extracted plantain leaf juice), and apply it to the affected skin. Keep it in place for an hour, and then wash it off with cool water. Repeat daily for a week.

Plantain leaf tincture

From fresh leaf:
> 4 ounces (100 g) fresh leaves
> 8 fluid ounces (200 ml) 190 proof
> grain alcohol (95%)

From dried leaf:
> 4 ounces (100 g) dried leaves
> 20 fluid ounces (500 ml) 120 proof
> grain alcohol (60%)

Put the herb in a glass jar, cover with alcohol, and close the lid tightly. Steep 2-4 weeks, strain, and bottle. Label (example, fresh: "Common plantain leaf, 1:2 95%, 7.2021, trail in the woods"; example, dried: "Ribwort plantain leaf, 1:5 60%, 12.2021, storebought").

Dosage is 15-40 drops, 1-3 times a day for earache, tinnitus, middle ear infection, sinusitis, or toothache.

Use the fresh leaf to treat acne.

Plantain stops bleeding. Apply a crushed fresh leaf to stop nosebleed, for example.

The juice from a crushed plantain leaf helps stop the necrosis of some spider bites, so keep some around if you live where venomous spiders are part of the local ecology.

Use a plantain leaf tincture for earache, tinnitus, middle ear infection or "glue ear," sinusitis, and toothache.

The seeds of various plantains have been used for centuries to relieve constipation. The seeds of even common plantain will work, although gathering the seeds is tedious and slow.

If you look for plantain seeds (also called ispaghula or psyllium seed) in your health food store, chose products that include no added sugar or contact laxatives. The seeds work because they're mucilaginous, so take them with plenty of water.

128

Plantain seed in water

1 tablespoon plantain (or ispaghula or psyllium) seed
1 cup (250 ml) cold water
unsweetened sour juice (optional)

Pour the herb in a glass, add water, and let it swell for 20 minutes. Stir, add sour juice such as currant or lingonberry if desired, and drink.

Chia seed (Salvia columbariae or Salvia hispanica) works the same way.

Plantain leaf syrup

Make a syrup from plantain leaf using the recipe on page 1.

Take a spoonful as needed for respiratory problems or a sore throat.

Plantain leaf oil and salve

Make an oil from dried leaf and make a salve from that (see recipe on page 7).

Use the salve for cuts, scrapes, bruises, and itchy insect bites.

FOOD USES

To use plantain leaf as a wild green, slice larger leaves crossways every ½ inch (1-2 cm) to cut through tough leaf veins. Smaller leaves can be used as they are.

Add younger, more tender leaves to salads and older, tougher leaves to stews and soups.

OTHER USES

Cage birds love plantain seeds. Gather entire flower stalks when the seeds are almost ripe and hang them in the cage.

WARNINGS

Plantain itself won't cause allergies, but pollen does fall on its broad, spread-out leaves from nearby trees and grasses. Avoid using plantain if you get pollen-related reactions from it.

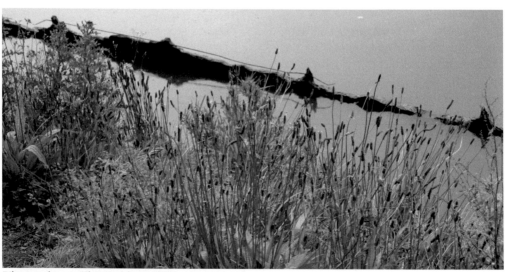

Ribwort plantain (Plantago lanceolata).

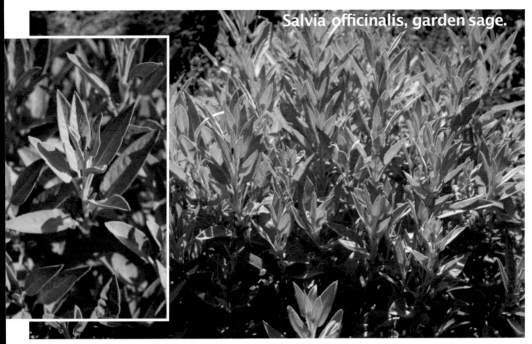

Salvia officinalis, garden sage.

SAGE

It either increases or reduces sweating and milk secretion.

Garden sage (Salvia officinalis), also called common sage.

Other useful aromatic and bitter Salvia species include:

- white sage (Salvia apiana), also called bee sage and sacred sage
- glutinous sage, sticky sage (Salvia glutinosa), also called Jupiter's sage
- woodland sage, Balkan clary (Salvia nemorosa)
- clary, clary sage (Salvia sclarea)

Note that sagebrushes and mugworts are not sages but are instead Artemisia species, and are not covered here.

Taste: Aromatic, bitter.

Energetics: Warming, drying.

Family: Mint family, Lamiaceae.

Perennial: Harvest from summer to fall. Clary sage is biennial.

Habitat: There are no wild sages in Finland.

Like most Mediterrannean plants, garden sage requires permeable soil, prefers lime over acidity, and likes full sun. ("Full sun" doesn't mean the same thing in Finland as it does in, say, Arizona.)

Don't plant your garden sage in clay if you want it to flourish and flower.

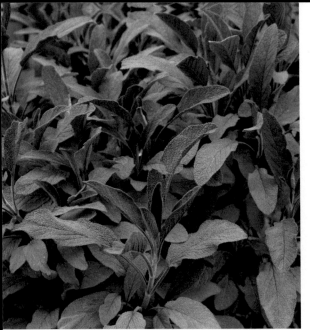

The purple–leafed cultivar of garden sage (Salvia officinalis 'Purpurascens').

Cultivation: Seeds or cuttings.

Garden sage is green year–round, so if you live in a cold climate, cover it in fall. Although uncovered sage will look fabulous when it first appears from beneath the snow in spring, because the ground is still frozen, it will soon die of thirst.

Make new plants from established garden sage by "layering": bend and pin long stems to the ground using a stone or other heavy object, and then wait for roots to form where the plant touches the soil. Once it has rooted, cut it away from the mother plant.

Garden sage cultivars include Salvia officinalis 'Icterina' with its yellow–green variegated leaves; 'Purpurascens' with purple leaves; 'Tricolor' with red–white–and–green variegated leaves; and 'Berggarten', which has very large green leaves. The cultivars are less hardy than regular garden sage. Propagate them from cuttings.

I've grown white sage (Salvia apiana) in my garden several times. It's at home in the mountains of southern California, but it doesn't survive Finland's long (long!) winters.)

Clary sage is a biennial. So far, it hasn't survived a winter in my garden.

Appearance: Garden sage is almost a groundcover here, but in warmer climates it can grow to 18 inches (50 cm) or taller. The leaf is a gray–green and hairy. The flower stalk with its blue blossoms rises out of the leaf mass.

Clary sage produces stunning flower spikes in its second year.

Important constituents: Garden sage contains essential oils (including thujone, borneol, and camphor), tannins (rosmarinic acid and similar caffeic acid derivatives), flavonoids, bitter substances, and a resin.

PICKING AND PROCESSING

Gather single leaves or cut twigs and branches from spring to fall. Cut the plant back to ground level in fall if you suspect winter will kill it.

Gather flowering stalks when the plant is in full flower.

Spread your harvest to dry or dry it in hanging bundles. You can also tincture the fresh herb.

Some people prefer the purple–leaf cultivar, but any sage works if it's an aromatic bitter one.

I save white sage for special occasions and for smudging. Its tincture also makes a nice perfume.

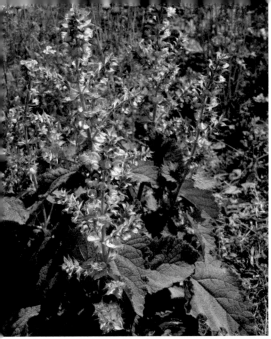
Clary sage (Salvia sclarea).

EFFECTS AND USES

Because sage is bitter, it strengthens appetite and digestion, especially of fatty foods. If you're always uncomfortable after eating fried food, spice it with sage—or take sage tincture or tea 20 minutes before your fatty meal.

Because sage is aromatic, it helps with mild digestive pain and menstrual cramps.

Use it for problems in the mouth and throat, such as hoarseness, sore throat, chafing dentures, and gum disease. Gargle with a cooled sage tea or spritz it into your mouth for these problems, as well as for the common cold.

Sage strengthens the lungs. Drink hot sage tea as needed for respiratory problems. If you catch every passing respiratory bug, drink hot sage tea thrice daily for a month or two. The sage tea treatment won't help if your lung problems are due to mold in your environment, however.

Sage is nicely twofold in its effect on sweating and milk secretion.

If you take your sage tea cold, or take your sage tincture in cold water, it will stop excessive sweating and reduce milk secretion. The effect of sage on sweating, when taken cold, is so reliable that menopausal ladies love this herb: it curbs hot flushes and night sweats.

If you sweat too much and aren't menopausal, visit a doctor to find out why.

Sage taken hot makes you sweat more, and it promotes milk production.

If you have low blood pressure and don't sweat enough (you can't handle hot weather, and a sauna is completely out of the question), you may be a "dry" person. In this case, sage is a poor choice. Use mucilaginous herbs, instead, such as marshmallow root or psyllium seed.

Sage calms and reduces nervousness and anxiety.

Because also helps memory, sage is especially good for students and the elderly. In this regard, though, it's useful for everyone. A cup of sage tea every day is enough. If you don't like the taste of sage, use rosemary, instead.

Sage tea
1-2 teaspoons dried or fresh sage
1 cup (250 ml) boiling water

Pour boiling water over the herb, steep 10 minutes, and strain.

Drink 1-3 cups a day cold to curb sweating or milk production. For other uses, drink the tea hot.

Lemon juice squeezed into your sage tea removes the bitterness.

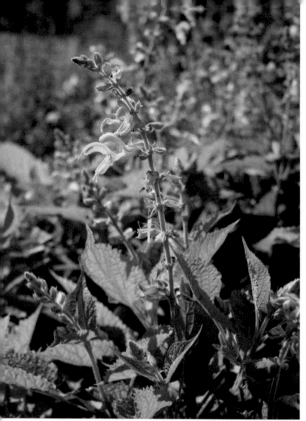

Glutinous sage (Salvia glutinosa).

Sage tincture

From fresh herb:
  4 ounces (100 g) fresh sage
  8 fluid ounces (200 ml) 190 proof
    grain alcohol (95%)

From dried herb:
  4 ounces (100 g) dried sage
  20 fluid ounces (500 ml) 120 proof
    grain alcohol (60%)

Put the herb in a glass jar, cover with the alcohol, and close the lid tightly. Steep 2–4 weeks, strain, and bottle. Label (example, fresh: "Glutinous sage, 1:2 95%, 8.2021, my garden"; example, dried: "White sage, 1:5 60%, 12.2021, gift from Ginia").

Dosage is 30–60 drops, 1–3 times a day.

To gargle, use a spoonful in a glass of warm water.

Sage wine

½ ounce (15 g) crushed dried sage
2 cups (500 ml) white or red wine

Put the herb in a glass jar, cover with the wine, and close the lid tightly. Leave for a week, shaking the jar from time to time. Strain through a coffee filter.

Take 2 tablespoons 3 times a day for nervousness and exhaustion.

Sage compress for sweaty hands and feet

a handful dried sage
  or two handfuls fresh
1 quart (1 l) water

Pour boiling water over the herb, steep 15 minutes, strain, and cool to just skin-comfortable. Dip a cloth in the tea, wring out the excess liquid, and apply it to sweating hands or feet for 30–40 minutes.

A sage bath

2 quarts (2 l) boiling water
dried or fresh sage
3 tablespoons kosher salt

Fresh herb: Cover herb with water.

Dried herb: Put herb in a pan and add triple the amount of water.

Bring to a boil, add the salt, turn off heat, and steep 15 minutes. Strain. Add to bathwater with enough cold water to make a comfortable bath. Get in and enjoy!

A sage bath is refreshing and warming.

FOOD USES

Sage goes well with greasy meats such as goose, lamb, mutton, and eel. Take care not to use too much, though; the strong flavor can overwhelm.

OTHER USES

Use sage to flavor your tooth powder.

Add sage to deodorant bags to reduce sweating

A strong sage tea enhances dark hair color.

Tooth powder

4 ounces (100 g) fresh sage, thyme, or mint
2 ounces (50 g) kosher salt

Grind dry ingredients into a fine powder. Store in an airtight jar.

Sprinkle a pinch of the powder on a moistened toothbrush instead of toothpaste.

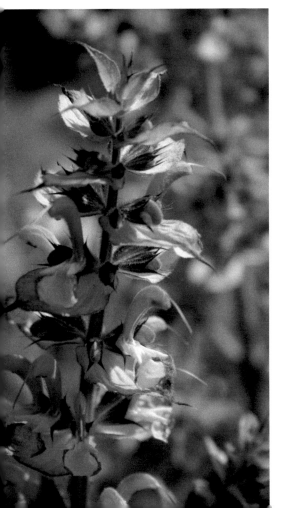

Deodorant powder

1 ounce (25 g) dried, powdered scented herbs, such as sage, thyme, lavender, rose, and/or mint
1 ounce (25 g) baking soda
6 ounces (150 g) potato starch
muslin cloth
string

Combine ingredients. Cut muslin cloth into 6-inch-square(15 cm) pieces. Put a tablespoon of the mix in the center of each square. Take each cloth by the corners, twirl it around once above the contents, and tie with some pretty string. Pat the pouch under your arms and in other sweating spots. Remember that the light-colored powder will be visible on dark clothing.

Keep the deodorant pouches in a plastic bag or a glass or plastic container, as the powder will leak.

Note: Because of its tiny particles, this deodorant mix is unsuitable for use by asthma sufferers.

WARNINGS

Avoid sage during pregnancy. Don't use it if you are nursing, either, unless you specifically need to reduce or increase your milk.

There's more thujone in the tincture than in the tea. Don't take more tincture than suggested.

Those suffering from epilepsy should use only small doses of sage, because of the thujone.

In rare instances, sage can cause a rash.

The stunning flower spike of clary sage.

PYRROLIZIDINE ALKALOIDS

Don't ingest plants that contain liver–toxic pyrrolizidine alkaloids.

Alkaloids are alkaline substances that have a variety of physiological effects on humans.

The alkaloids caffeine, nicotine, and morphine, for instance, have strong effects.

Berberine is a mild alkaloid that strengthens liver function.

Some alkaloids don't affect us at all.

Pyrrolizidine alkaloids can be either liver–toxic or harmless.

Liver–toxic pyrrolizidine alkaloids occur in herbs such as comfrey (Symphytum spp.) and coltsfeet (Tussilago and Petasites spp.). All species of comfrey contain them, even yellow–and white–flowering species.

Echinacea species' pyrrolizidine alkaloids, on the other hand, are harmless.

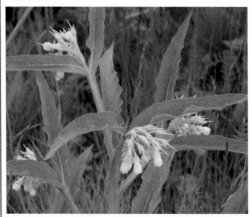

Comfrey (Symphytum officinale) contains liver-toxic pyrrolizidine alkaloids.

Liver–toxic pyrrolizidines cause a slow loss of liver function. You won't feel pain in your liver when you take coltsfoot or comfrey internally. Instead, your general well–being will decline gradually as liver damage accrues over time.

Veno–occlusive liver disease (which requires biopsy or autopsy to diagnose) can result from high–dose chemotherapy, heriditary immunodeficiency, or consumption of liver–toxic pyrrolizidine alkaloids.

Prior to a century ago no one knew about veno–occlusive liver disease, so no one suspected liver problems could result from using plants with liver–toxic pyrrolizidines.

Pyrrolizidine liver damage is insidious; you can't see cause and effect. And not everyone gets liver damage from eating the toxic plants.

The probability of liver damage is greater in "innocent" livers: fetuses, babies, and children are most vulnerable to toxic pyrrolizidines. Don't consume plants that contain liver–toxic pyrrolizidines if you're pregnant or nursing, and never give them to children.

Adults can make up their own minds on the matter, as long as they acknowledge the risks.

I strongly suggest only using these plants externally. We have plenty of risk–free herbal cough remedies and remedies for broken bones.

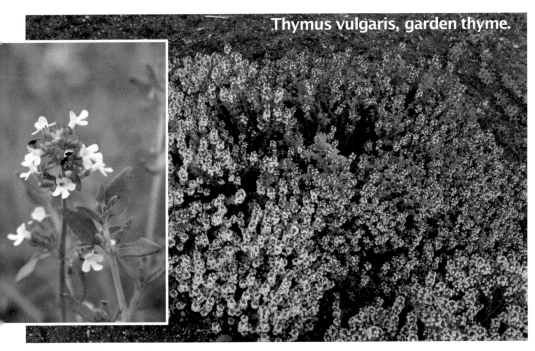

Thymus vulgaris, garden thyme.

THYME

Great for coughs and to aid digestion

Thymus species include

- Garden thyme (Thymus vulgaris); also called common thyme, English thyme, French thyme, summer thyme, winter thyme
- Breckland thyme, wild thyme (Thymus serpyllum); also called creeping thyme, lavender thyme, mother of thyme
- Large thyme (Thymus pulegioides); also called greater wild thyme, wild thyme
- Lemon thyme (Thymus ×citriodorus)

Other thymes work, as well, but try to use those with the same heat as garden thyme.

Taste: Aromatic, from mildly spicy to fiery.

Energetics: Heating or warming, drying.

Family: Mint family, Lamiaceae.

Perennial: Harvest from summer to fall.

Habitat: Wild thymes thrive in permeable soil in sunny spots. You'll find them on sandy beaches and gravelly ridges. They're easiest to spot in the beginning of July, when they flower in colorful ground-huggingsplashes.

Cultivation: Sow the seeds outdoors in fall or spring. Ground-hugging thymes also grow well from runners.

A flowering mat of groundcover thymes can range in color from white to deep purple.

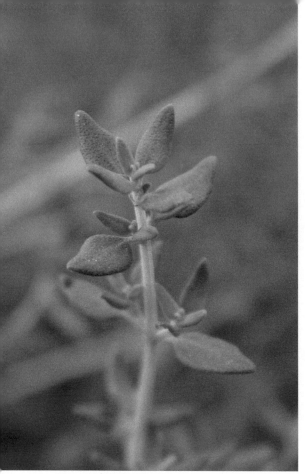

Leaves of garden thyme.

Thymes hybridize easily, so botanical names are seldom very reliable. Choose plants based on scent or growth habit instead of species, cultivar, or hybrid name.

Thymes are evergreen plants, appearing from beneath the snow in spring looking robust healthy. Unfortunately, a large part of the plant often dies when the sun shines warmly while the ground is still frozen, so cover your thyme plants before winter snows arrive. Garden thyme and other thymes with an upright growth habit are most vulnerable; they won't sprout roots everywhere a branch touches soil, as groundcovers do.

Appearance: Thyme leaves are oval. Garden thyme leaves may appear to be diamond-shaped, but if you flatten them you'll see that they, too, are oval.

Flower color varies from white to deep purple. Thyme plants are quite showy in full flower. In good years, blossoms can completely obscure the foliage.

Important constituents: Thymes contain essential oils (thymol, carvacrol), tannins, and bitter substances.

PICKING AND PROCESSING

Cut the top off thymes either in full flower or in fall. At other times you won't get as much herb for your trouble then.

Spread thymes that have woody stems to dry completely; then put them into a paper bag and shake the bag gently to loosen the leaves. If you're too rough, you'll end up with woody twig bits in your dried leaf.

Remove the largest stems and pour the leaf and remaining few twig bits into a glass jar.

Make a syrup, honey, or tincture from the fresh tops, or use them in cooking.

EFFECTS AND USES

Garden thyme (Thymus vulgaris) is best for medicinal uses.

The other thymes are useful in proportion to their heat. If you don't have a hot thyme, you can use milder species, but they won't be as effective.

Thymes are anti-inflammatory and tasty. I often add them to otherwise bad-tasting tea blends.

Thymes strengthen the lungs.

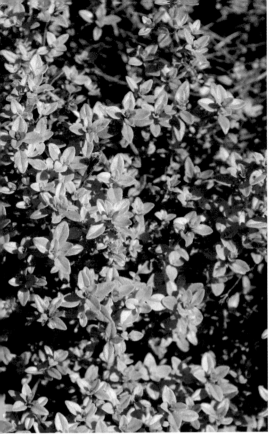

Golden-leafed lemon thyme in early summer (Thymus ×citriodorus).

If you catch every cold or cough making the rounds, drink thyme or sage (Salvia spp.) tea regularly.

Also use thyme for a sudden cough or for bronchitis, sore throat, and hoarseness.

Thymes are excellent when a cough is about to end and phlegm turns tough and dry.

Try to drink enough hot thyme tea to make your breath smell of thyme. A cup or two a day will help some, but in this instance more is better.

Use thyme for gut upset, diarrhea, loss of appetite, and gas and bloating.

Thyme is ideal for nausea, as well. It's almost as good as ginger, if you're not a "hot" person.

If you drink a thyme tea sweetened with honey after partying heavily but before bed, your hangover will be less severe. Thyme tea can also help in the morning, both for nausea and for headache.

Use lukewarm thyme tea to wash small wounds and scrapes.

Make a thyme bath for coughs, colds, and joint pain.

Thymes can be used like beebalms, as well (see page 30).

Thyme tea

1 teaspoon thyme
1 cup (250 ml) boiling water

Pour boiling water over the herb and steep 5-10 minutes. Don't let this tea steep too long! Strain and drink one to three cups a day.

Sweeten your tea with sugar or honey for respiratory problems, but leave it unsweetened if you're taking it for digestive upset.

For a sore throat and hoarseness, you can also pour some tea into a small spray bottle and mist the back of your throat with it.

Thyme honey

Refer to the recipe on page 2, or make thyme honey like this:
½ounce (15 g) dried thyme
10-18 ounces (300-500 g) organic honey

Pour herb and honey into a jar, lid tightly, and leave the mix for 2-6 weeks. Then either remove the thyme from the top of the honey (storing it in another jar to use, as well), or leave it as is.

Take a spoonful as needed.

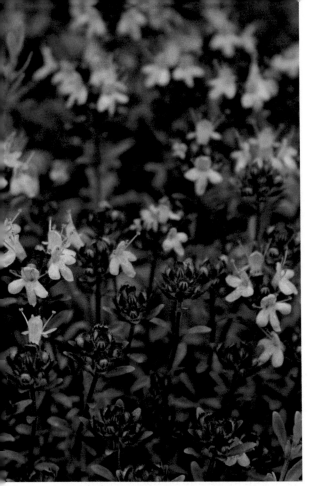

The flowers of wild thyme (Thymus serpyllum).

Thyme syrup

Make a syrup using the recipe on page 1.

Take spoonful of syrup as needed for cough or sore throat.

Thyme tincture

From fresh herb:
  4 ounces (100 g) fresh herb, in ½–to
    1–inch(1–3 cm) pieces
  8 fluid ounces (200 ml) 190 proof grain
    alcohol (95%)

From dried herb:
  4 ounces (100 g) dried herb
  20 fluid ounces (500 ml) 120 proof grain
    alcohol (60%)

Put the herb in a glass jar, cover with the alcohol, and close the lid tightly. Steep two to four weeks, strain and bottle. Label (example, fresh: "Thyme, 1:2 95%, 6.2021, my garden"; example, dried: "Large thyme, 1:5 60%, 12.2021, Granddad's garden").

Dosage is 15–30 drops 1–3 times a day.

A thyme footbath

  1 quart (1 l) boiling water
  1 cup (250 ml) fresh or dried thyme
  3 tablespoons kosher or sea salt

Put the herb in a pan, and add water and salt. Bring to a boil, steep for 15 minutes, and strain. Pour into a basin or large bowl and add cold water to cool to a comfortable temperature. Soak your feet 10–20 minutes. Very enjoyable!

A thyme bath

  2 quarts (2 l) boiling water
  dried or fresh thyme

Fresh herb: Cover herb with water.

Dried herb: Put herb in a pan and add triple the amount of water.

Bring to a boil, turn off heat, and steep for 15 minutes. Strain. Pour into bathwater and add enough cold water to make for a comfortable bath. Get in and enjoy!

A thyme bath is good for coughs or joint pain and helps strengthen the system against flu.

FOOD USES

Thyme is an important culinary herb, prominent in both bouquet garni and herbes de Provence.

A bouquet garni starts with thyme and bay leaf, with herbs such as sage, parsley, rosemary, oregano, marjoram, and basil, added according to preference. Tie up the bundle with a length of heavy cotton string.

Herbes de Provence blends various dried herbs. Try this combination: 1 teaspoon each thyme, sage, savory, and rosemary, ½ teaspoon each oregano or marjoram and basil, and a pinch of lavender or fennel seed.

OTHER USES

Use lukewarm thyme tea as a face wash.

WARNINGS

Avoid the thymes if they give you a rash.

Don't use thyme in large amounts if you are pregnant or breastfeeding.

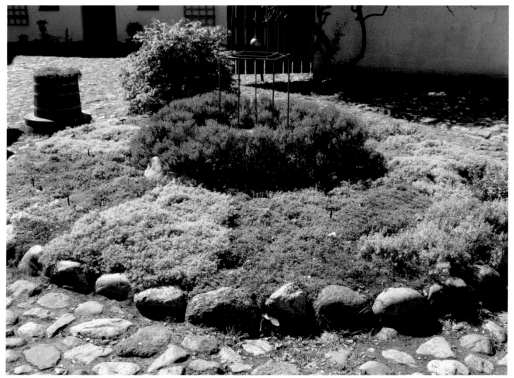

Various ground-covering thymes surround upright garden thyme in this attractive planting at Tirups Herb Garden near Lund in Sweden.

CUCUMBER AND ITS USES

Cucumbers cool and refresh, and they're nutrient-rich.

Raw cucumber is perfect to eat as-is or in salads on hot summer days, but did you know you can juice up winter stews with cucumber cubes?

Cucumbers contain a lot of water. Those grown in rich soil will also contain calcium, magnesium, and potassium.

Cukes are high in flavonoids, beta-carotene, and vitamins B (B1, B5, B6), C, and K.

Most of these nutrients are stored in the skin and seeds. Use organically grown cucumbers so you can eat the skin.

Fresh cucumber slices cool and soothe sunburn and similarly hot and red skin problems.

Held in the mouth, a bit of cucumber helps with halitosis due to mouth bacteria. (Peppermint helps with bacteria in the esophagus. If the smell sits still deeper, support the liver with herbs such as yellow dock or dandelion.)

Cucumber slices revitalize tired eyes, but don't touch the side of the slice that lies against the lids.

Cucumber oil and salve

First make an oil from grated cucumber, and then use the oil to make a salve (see recipe on page 7).

Use oil or salve for itch or for aggressive red eczema.

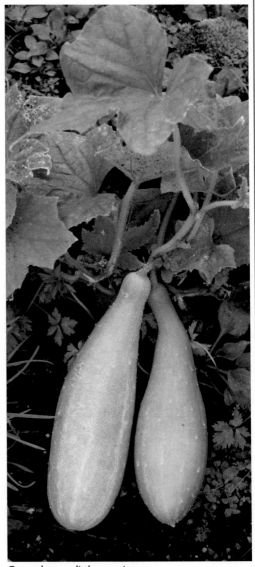

Cucumbers, a little overripe.

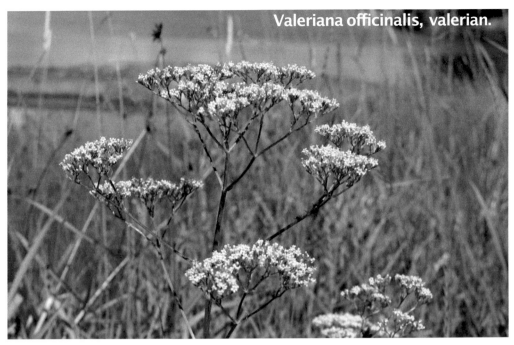

Valeriana officinalis, valerian.

VALERIAN

Calming for the cool, not so for the hot.

Valeriana species: Including
- valerian (Valeriana officinalis), also called garden valerian
- common valerian (Valeriana sambucifolia)

Valerians do hybridize.

Taste: Aromatic.

Energetics: Warming, drying.

Family: Valerian family, Valerianaceae. Also honeysuckle family, Caprifoliaceae.

Perennial: Harvest the root in autumn. Aboveground parts can be harvested in summer.

Habitat: Valerian thrives in moist spots. Look for it in ditches and along lakeshores and riverbanks.

Cultivation: Sow seeds outdoors in fall or spring. Leave the seeds uncovered.

In fertile garden soil, valerian grows up to 9 feet (3 m) tall! It will fall over in strong winds, and it self-seeds profusely. In the wild, valerian usually tops out at around 3 feet (1 m).

Appearance: Valerian leaves and flower stems grow from a small root clump. The flowers are white or light pink, and their scent is overwhelming.

Seen from afar, the flower heads form easily recognized triangular arcs.

The leaves are pinnate; that is, they come in pairs with an end leaflet.

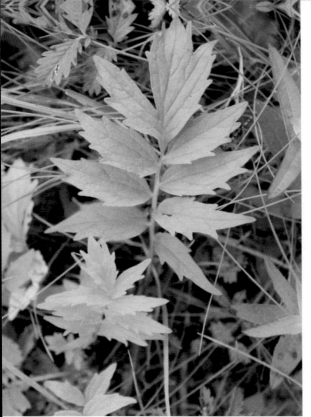

The leaf of common valerian (Valeriana sambucifolia).

The leaflets of garden valerian are all the same size. Common valerian's end leaflet is much larger than the others.

Valerian roots are short, with individual root thickness measuring usually around 1/8-inch(3 mm). (It's amazing the plant can stay upright.)

Important constituents: Valerian contains valepotriates, alkaloids, flavonoids, and an essential oil with sesquiterpenes (valerenic acid).

PICKING AND PROCESSING

Use a shovel to dig valerian root in the fall or late summer.

If valerian grows in a boggy (but not grass–covered) spot, you can do without the shovel. Grasp firmly the plant's

leaves and flower stalks close to the ground, and pull upward with a gentle shaking motion.

Wash the roots.

If you plan to dry your valerian roots, keep housecats out of the drying room or away from your dehydrator.

Fresh roots can be tinctured.

Store dried valerian roots in airtight glass jars. The longer the root is in the jar, the stronger the scent. Use dried root in teas or tinctures.

Aboveground valerian parts are best harvested during or before flowering. Cut the material into inch–long(3 cm) pieces and spread them to dry. Cats are less interested in aboveground valerian, but the scent of the flowers soon induces headache.

Store dried valerian in airtight glass jars. Use it in teas, make it into tinctures, or chew on a bit of leaf or stem as needed.

It doesn't matter whether the flower is white or pink.

Most valerian species are about equally strong and can be used interchangeably.

EFFECTS AND USES

Use valerian root or aboveground parts, fresh or dry.

The root is stronger than the aboveground parts. Dry is stronger than fresh.

Valerian is a well–known sleeping aid. For instance, it's great if you need to go to sleep early in the evening. A cup of valerian tea at 6:00, half a cup at 7:00, and another half–cup when you go to bed at 7:30 virtually guarantees sleep.

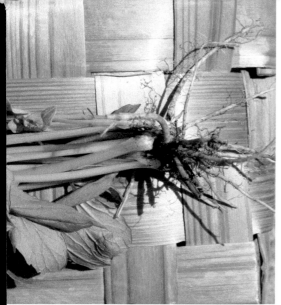

Valerian root.

Valerian isn't suitable for "hot" people—those who wear T-shirtswhen everyone else is wearing sweaters. Although they'll sleep very well with valerian's help, they'll awaken feeling bone-tired and worn out.

Valerian's probably not a good idea to treat long-term insomnia. Instead, find the reason for the sleeplessness and do something about that.

Although valerian can be useful for menstrual pain and muscle cramps, magnesium and vitamin B are better.

A mild valerian tea helps with headaches and nerve pain.

Valerian is good for anxiety and fears, and for the nervousness that stress brings. For these, use it as a bath or make a mild tea—a cold maceration of the root or a normal tea of aboveground parts. Take magnesium and vitamin B, as well.

A valerian bath helps relieve joint and muscle pains. If you take a valerian bath in the evening, you'll relax and sleep well.

Valerian

Valerian tea

1-2 teaspoons dried or fresh valerian root
1 cup (250 ml) boiling water

Pour boiling water over the root, steep 10 minutes, and strain.

Drink a cupful 2 hours before bedtime, half a cup an hour before bedtime, and another half-cup at bedtime.

Don't use valerian regularly to treat insomnia. Instead, address the cause of the sleeplessness.

Valerian maceration

1-2 teaspoons dried valerian root
1 cup (250 ml) cold water

Steep the dried root in the cold water 4-12 hours, and then strain.

Drink 1-2 cups a day.

A valerian maceration is mild and helps headaches, nervousness, and nerve pain.

Valerian tincture

From fresh root:
4 ounces (100 g) fresh root
8 fluid ounces (200 ml) 190 proof
grain alcohol (95%)

From dried herb:
4 ounces (100 g) dried root or aboveground parts
20 fluid ounces (500 ml) 120 proof
grain alcohol (60%)

Put the root in a glass jar, cover with the alcohol, and close the lid tightly. Steep 2-4 weeks, strain, bottle, and label (example, fresh: "Valerian root, 1:2 95%, 7.2021, by the brook"; example, dried: "Valerian root, 1:5 60%, 12.2021, watery meadow").

Dosage is 30-90 drops as needed. Don't use valerian every day.

A valerian bath

  2 quarts (2 l) boiling water
  dried or fresh aboveground parts of valerian

Fresh herb: Cover herb with water.

Dried herb: Put herb in a pan and add triple the amount of water.

Bring to a boil, turn off heat, and steep for 15 minutes. Strain. Add to bathwater with enough cold water to make a comfortable bath. Get in and enjoy!

This bath is relaxing.

A valerian root bath

  1 quart (1 liter) boiling water
  4 ounces (100 g) fresh valerian root

Pour the water over the root and steep 10 hours. Strain and add to bathwater with enough warm water to make a comfortable bath. Get in and enjoy!

This bath is relaxing and reduces joint pain.

OTHER USES

Make a cat toy from valerian root—but make sure it's sturdy!

Or stuff fresh valerian roots in an old heavy sock and tie the end. As the roots dry, some (not all) cats will enjoy chewing it to bits.

It's believed that cats go wild over valerian because the scent resembles cat sex pheromones. This is false advertising—unfair!

WARNINGS

Don't use valerian if you're a "hot" person. Instead, use California poppy (Eschscholzia californica) for sleeplessness.

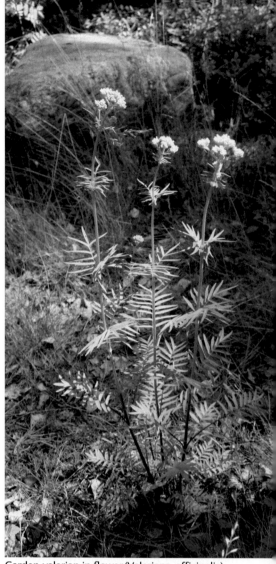

Garden valerian in flower (Valeriana officinalis).

Avoid valerian if you use calming or antidepressive medicines or take sleeping pills.

Large amounts of valerian can cause depression and headache in some people.

Valerian can cause palpitations. If you react this way, stop taking valerian.

145

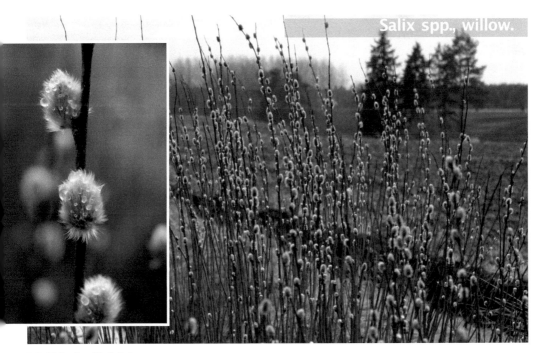

Salix spp., willow.

WILLOW

Willow soothes pain. Its catkins calm overactive sex hormones.

Salix species.

Taste: Bitter, astringent.

Energetics: Cooling, drying.

Family: Willow family, Salicaceae.

Perennial: Harvest willow catkins and bark in spring and leaf in summer.

Habitat: Most willows thrive in damp places.

Cultivation: Cut willow twigs or small branches root easily in spring and early summer.

Species with long straight branches, such as common osier (Salix viminalis) and purple osier or purple willow (Salix purpurea), can be grown as a woven hedge or in rows. The year's long shoots are cut in fall for use in basketry.

Some willows (the weeping willows, for instance) are grown as ornamental trees.

Appearance: In early spring, many willows have silvery, smooth catkins or flower buds.

Male and female flowers blossom on separate plants. The male catkins release pollen, and the females release fluffy ripe seed later on.

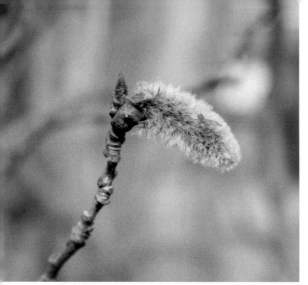

The silvery flower bud of European aspen (Populus tremula).

Look–alikes: Flower buds of some poplars and aspens are also soft and silvery, but they grow on small concentrated spurs. Although these catkins aren't toxic, I don't know whether they can be used as one would willow catkins.

Important constituents: The action of willow derives from its salicylates and tannins.

PICKING AND PROCESSING

Gather willow catkins in spring. They start out very small, growing larger and larger from week to week. I've picked them as tiny silvery nubbins and as yellowing catkins of either gender.

If you wait to pick your catkins until after the flowers start to turn yellow, your basket will fill in no time. They'll be 1–2½ inches (3–7 cm) long and fully grown. "Milking" the willow branches and twigs works best for this.

If you pick only the silvery pretty things, count on filling a small tincture jar a half–inch at a time. Cover each addition with your choice of alcohol.

Fresh willow catkins are very effective for calming excessive reproductive hormones in both males and females.

Strip the bark in spring, when it's easy to separate from the wood. If barking season is over by the time you get to a willow stand, chop the twigs into ½–1-inch (1–3 cm) lengths and use those, instead.

Harvest the leaves in summer.

You may dry leaf, bark, or twig pieces, or use them fresh.

EFFECTS AND USES

Willow catkin tincture curbs excessive production of reproductive hormones.

Teens will notice they're better able to control their hormones, instead of the hormones controlling them.

Taking willow catkin tincture can even regulate the inordinate sexual desires of some adults.

The tincture also helps to even out the hormonal rollercoaster of menopause.

Use willow bark or twig bits in oils, salves, poultices, and baths for aches and pains in muscles and joints. I don't recommend using them as a tea: it tastes ghastly, and the combined tannins and salicylates irritate tender guts.

Willow catkin tincture

4 ounces (100 g) fresh catkins
8 fluid ounces (200 ml) 190 proof grain alcohol (95%)

Put catkins in a glass jar, cover with alcohol, and close the lid tightly. Steep 2–4 weeks, strain, and bottle. Label (example: "Willow catkins, 1:2 95%, 5.2021, nearby marshes").

Dosage is 10–60 drops, 3–4 times a day.

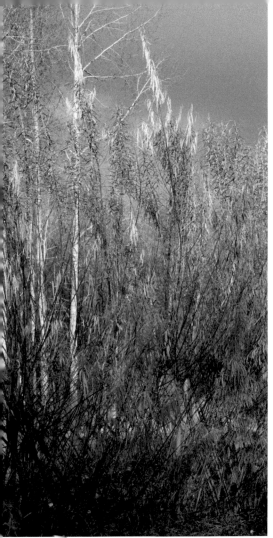

By autumn, a woven willow hedge is many yards (meters) tall.

A willow bath

water
dried or fresh willow leaf, bark or twigs

Fresh herb: Add herb to a pan with water to cover.

Dried herb: Put herb in a pan with three times as much water.

Bring to a boil, turn off heat, and steep 15 minutes. Strain. Add to bathwater with enough cold water to make a comfortable bath.

Get in and enjoy!

This is very good for the all-over ache you get after a thorough workout you're not yet accustomed to.

Willow oil and salve

Make an oil from dried bark, leaf, or twigs and make a salve from that (refer to the recipe on page 7).

Apply it for aches and pains.

Willow compress

1 handful dried willow leaf or bark
    or two handfuls fresh
1 quart (1 l) water

Pour boiling water over the herb, steep 15 minutes, strain, and cool to just skin-comfortable. Dip a cloth in the tea, and then squeeze out the excess liquid.

Put the moist, hot cloth on the achy spot and leave it there 30–40 minutes.

OTHER USES

Use willow twigs to hold up garden peas (but remember that willows root easily).

In spring, use willows to make your own rooting hormone: put a handful of chopped willow twigs in a glass of water along with cuttings of other plants. The cuttings will root before too long.

Long, straight willow shoots are used in basketry.

WARNINGS

Those sensitive to salicylates shouldn't use willow.

I recommend against using willow bark, leaf, or twig internally, because they can irritate stomach lining. I much prefer meadowsweet for internal use.

LILY FLOWER AND ITS USES

Lilies are both pretty and medicinal.

Use only true lilies (Lilium spp.). I use a tincture made from only the fresh flowers. Any color flower will work.

Lily flower tincture stimulates pelvic lymph flow, so it's good for some cysts.

Take lily flower tincture for infertility if you also suffer from polycystic ovary syndrome (PCOS), or from metabolic syndrome.

Lily flower will bring on balky menses when you constantly feel as if it's just around the corner. (Do first check that you're not pregnant, though!)

Use the tincture if your menses flow only when you walk and not when you sit or stand.

Take the tincture when you have an ache or a stabbing pain in your uterus.

Give the tincture a try for prolapsed uterus. It works if the uterus is heavy with fibroids.

In large amounts, lily flower tincture can cause nausea, vomiting, and diarrhea. Don't take more than the suggested dosage!

Lily flower tincture

    4 ounces (100 g) fresh lily flowers without
        green parts
    8 fluid ounces (200 ml) 190 proof
        grain alcohol (95%)

Put the flowers in a glass jar, cover with the alcohol, and close the lid tightly. Steep 2-4 weeks, strain, and bottle.

Label (example: "Madonna lily, 1:2 95%, 7.2021, my garden").

Dosage is 1-5 drops, 1-3 times a day. Don't take more than this!

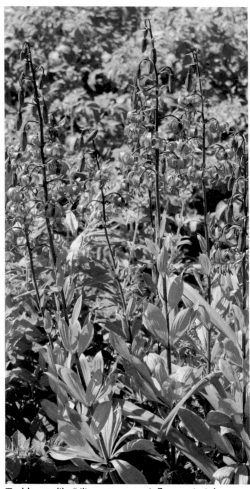

Turk's-cap lily (Lilium martagon) flowers in July.

Index